NEH

Fulbright Papers

PROCEEDINGS OF COLLOQUIA

SPONSORED BY THE
UNITED STATES–UNITED KINGDOM
EDUCATIONAL COMMISSION:
THE FULBRIGHT COMMISSION, LONDON

Volume 15

Life and death under high technology medicine

The major social and cultural consequences of recent developments in high technology medicine are just as profound as the ethical implications which have dominated the debate to date.

The contributors to this volume, who include clinicians, social scientists, lawyers and philosophers, reflect on how developments at the frontiers of medicine are challenging our ideas about when life begins and ends, and about the possibilities in between. They explore how the 'new genetics' is challenging our understanding of what constitutes kinship, and how organ transplantations are shifting the boundaries between life and death. The emergence of an increasing range of ethical dilemmas for individuals is just part of the story; we also need to re-examine the consequences of high technology medicine for our understanding of the nature of social life and our cultural identity.

The Fulbright Programme of Educational Exchanges, which has been in operation since 1946, aims to promote mutual understanding between the United States of America and other nations. It now operates in more than 120 countries, with forty-three bi-national commissions involved in its administration. In the United Kingdom the Commission aims to offer qualified British and American nationals the opportunity to exchange significant knowledge and educational experience in fields of consequence to the two countries, and thereby to contribute to a deeper mutual understanding of Anglo-American relations and to broaden the means by which the two societies can further their understanding of each other's cultures. Amongst its activities the Commission promotes annual colloquia on topics of Anglo-American interest; the proceedings are published in this series.

Life and death under high technology medicine

edited by
IAN ROBINSON

MANCHESTER
UNIVERSITY PRESS

IN ASSOCIATION WITH
THE FULBRIGHT COMMISSION, LONDON

DISTRIBUTED EXCLUSIVELY IN THE USA AND CANADA
BY ST. MARTIN'S PRESS

COPYRIGHT © THE US–UK EDUCATIONAL COMMISSION 1994

Published by Manchester University Press
Oxford Road, Manchester M13 9NR, UK
and Room 400, 175 Fifth Avenue, New York, NY 10010, USA
in association with The Fulbright Commission,
6 Porter Street, London W1M 2HR, UK

Distributed exclusively in the USA and Canada by
St. Martin's Press, Inc., 175 Fifth Avenue, New York, NY 10010, USA

British Library Cataloguing-in-Publication Data
A catalogue record for this book is available from the British Library

Library of Congress Cataloging-in-Publication Data
Life and death under high technology medicine / edited by Ian
    Robinson
        p.   cm.—(Fulbright papers : v. 15)
    Includes index.
    Proceedings of a colloquium sponsored by the U.S.–U.K. Educational
Commission.
    ISBN 0–7190–3590–2 (hardback)
    1. Medical technology—Moral and ethical aspects—Congresses.
    2. Medical innovations—Moral and ethical aspects—Congresses.
    I. Robinson, Ian, 1943–.   II. United States-United Kingdom
Educational Commission.   III. Series.
    [DNLM: 1. Ethics, Medical—congresses.   2. Technology, High-Cost-
congresses.   W 50 L7218 1994]
    R855.3.L54   1994
    174'.2—dc20
    DNLM/DLC
    for Library of Congress   94–17574

ISBN 0–7190–3590–2 *hardback*

Phototypeset by Intype, London
Printed and bound in Great Britain
by Biddles Limited, Guildford and King's Lynn

Contents

Contributors

DAVID ARMSTRONG, Reader, Department of General Practice, United Medical and Dental Schools, Guy's Hospital, London, UK

MARTIN BOBROW, Prince Philip Professor of Paediatric Research, Paediatric Research Unit, United Medical and Dental Schools, Guy's Hospital, London, UK

MICHAEL CALNAN, Professor of the Sociology of Health, and Director, Centre for Health Services Studies, University of Kent, UK

CHARLES A. ERIN, Lecturer in Applied Psychology, Centre for Social Ethics and Policy, University of Manchester, UK

RONALD FRANKENBERG, Research Professor, Department of Sociology and Social Anthropology, University of Keele and Professor Associate, Department of Human Sciences, at Brunel, University of West London, UK

MICHAEL FREEMAN, Professor of Law, Department of Laws, University College, London, UK

JO GREEN, Senior Research Fellow, Centre for Family Studies, University of Cambridge, UK

JOHN HARRIS, Professor of Applied Philosophy, Centre for Social Ethics and Policy, University of Manchester, UK

ROGER HIGGS, Director and Professor of General Practice, Department of General Practice and Primary Care, King's College Medical and Dental School, University of London, UK

BRYAN JENNETT, Professor of Neurosurgery, Institute of Neurological Sciences, University of Glasgow, UK

REGINA KENEN, Associate Professor, Department of Sociology and Anthropology, Trenton State College, USA

MARGARET LOCK, Professor of Medical Anthropology, Department of Humanities and Social Studies in Medicine, McGill University, Canada

MARGOT LYON, Lecturer, Department of Prehistory and Anthropology, Australian National University, Australia

ELIZABETH MANNERS, Researcher, Paediatric Research Unit, United Medical and Dental Schools, Guy's Hospital, London, UK

THOMAS PRESTON, Chief, Cardiology Division, Pacific Medical Centre and Professor of Medicine, School of Medicine, University of Washington, Seattle, USA

MARTIN RICHARDS, Reader in Child Development, Centre for Family Studies, University of Cambridge, UK

IAN ROBINSON, Director, Centre for the Study of Health, Sickness and Disablement, Brunel, University of West London, UK

MARILYN STRATHERN, Professor of Social Anthropology, Department of Anthropology, University of Cambridge, UK

SIMON WILLIAMS, Lecturer, Department of Sociology, The University of Warwick, UK

Foreword

This volume records the proceedings of the Fulbright Colloquium on Life and Death under High Technology Medicine which was held at Brunel, The University of West London. The impact of modern medicine on the span of human life and on the choices now open at conception and birth is profound. The proposal made by the Centre for the Study of Health, Sickness and Disablement at Brunel University to mount an Anglo-American Colloquium to explore the social, legal and ethical issues involved was warmly welcomed by the Fulbright Commission which believes that, in this most important area, much of great value can be learnt from comparing views from both sides of the Atlantic.

In meeting its aim of promoting Anglo-American cultural understanding, the Commission sponsors at least one, and sometimes two, colloquia each year on subjects of mutual interest and importance to the United States and the United Kingdom. These meetings of distinguished scholars and practitioners in specialist fields augment the Commission's traditional awards of studentships, scholarships and fellowships to British and American citizens for study, teaching, research or work experience in the other's country. Over 11,000 such exchanges have been supported in this way by the Commission since it was established in 1948.

The Colloquium at Brunel covered a wide range of topics dealing with the impact of high technology medicine. Scholars and professional practitioners from the United Kingdom and the United States were joined by those from Canada and Australia to engage in discussions covering the many vital, controversial and fundamental issues involved.

The opinions expressed are, of course, personal to the contributors and do not necessarily reflect the views of the Commission. Nevertheless, the Commission believes that publication of the proceedings will be greatly valued by those working in the field of high technology medicine whilst at the same time be of special interest to all those concerned over the special effect this is having on our ways of thinking about life and death. The pace of change is accelerating and both the United Kingdom and the United States are in the forefront of new scientific developments and new approaches to the social and legal consequences of high technology medicine. The Fulbright Commission is pleased to have been able to contribute to its discussion at this time.

John E. Franklin, Executive Director
United States-United Kingdom Educational Commission
The Fulbright Commission, London

Acknowledgements

I acknowledge with grateful thanks the financial support of the Fulbright Commission for the Symposium on which this collection is based. Captain Franklin, Executive Director of the Commission, has been particularly helpful at all stages in planning and holding the Symposium, and in relation to the compilation of this collection following the meeting.

In addition to the contributors to this volume, I particularly wish to acknowledge the thoughtful criticisms and commentary of Meg Stacey during the Symposium on which this volume was based, from which I and other contributors gained considerably, and also to acknowledge the contribution of Mary-Jo Del Vecchio Good to the Symposium and its success.

In relation to the organisation of the meeting itself I am especially grateful for the individual administrative work of Jenny Charteris, for the secretarial support of Chris Alport, and for Margaret Hunter's contribution in making the meeting a success. Shirine Peseshgí played an important role in recording and annotating discussions at the Symposium, and at various points in my introduction I have drawn on her notes of the proceedings.

Abbreviations

ACMC	Andean Common Market and Community
AID	Artificial Insemination by Donor
AIDS	Acquired Immune Deficiency Syndrome
AFP	alpha-fetoprotein
ASEAN	Association of South East Asian Nations
BACUP	British Association of Cancer United Patients
CACM	Central American Common Market
CARICOM	Caribbean Economic Community
CCU	Coronary Care Unit
CEAO	Communauté Economique de l'Afrique de l'Ouest
CHD	coronary heart disease
CT	Computerised Tomography
CVS	chorionic villus sampling
DI	donor insemination
DIW	diseased in waiting
DNA	deoxyribonucleic acid
DOE	Department of Energy
EAO	East-African Community
EC	European Community
ECOWAS	Economic Community of West African States
ELSI	Ethical, Legal and Social Implications
ESRC	Economic and Science Research Council
FDA	Food and Drug Administration
FES	functional electrical stimulation
FNS	functional neuromuscular stimulation
HCL	hairy cell leukaemia
HFA	Human Fertilisation and Embryology
HGI	Human Genome Initiative
HGP	Human Genome Project
HIV	Human Immuno-deficiency Virus
HUGO	Human Genome Organization
ICU	Intensive Care Unit
IRB	Institutional Review Board
ISNIM	International Society for Neuroimmunomodulation
JMA	Japan Medical Association
LAFTA	Latin American Free Trade Association
MRI	Magnetic Resonance Imaging
NEI	neuro-endorcrinoimmunology

NIM	neuroimmunomodulation
NCHGR	National Centre for Human Genome Research
NHS	National Health Service
NIH	National Institutes of Health
PNI	psychoneuroimmunology
PPD	possibly, potentially diseased
PTCA	percutaneal transluminal coronary angioplasty
QALY	quality-adjusted life-year
UAE	United Arab Emirates
UCLA	University of California at Los Angeles
UDEAC	Union Douanière et Economique de l'Afrique
VAT	Value Added Tax

Introduction: Life and death under high technology medicine

IAN ROBINSON

There have always been technologies – drugs, devices, surgical and other procedures, and their support systems (Banta 1983) – associated with the management of health problems, and later with formal medical care. Many (perhaps most) of these technologies have started their lives as experimental creations in one form or another (Reiser 1978). Their transmutation into routine instruments of clinical practice has often occurred through unanticipated routes, which have owed more to the social, economic and cultural circumstances in which they were developed than to any intrinsic quality that they possessed (Bell 1989; Dominguez *et al.* 1987; Roth and Ruzek 1986; Scott 1990). However now we appear to be at a time in Europe and the United States when there is a striking emphasis on the more systematic development and evaluation of sophisticated technologies to assist, and sometimes to transform, certain medical practices managing life and death (Bijker, *et al.*1987; Foote 1987; Institute of Medicine 1985; Rublee 1989; Stocking 1982).

'High technology medicine' is an elusive phrase to define. For many, images of high technology medicine are indeed associated with novel, sophisticated and expensive kinds of medical equipment developed at the frontiers of scientific knowledge, and used to manage the frontiers of human life and death (Gabe and Calnan 1989). For others however the settings in which the equipment is placed – the operating theatre or the intensive care unit, and its style of use – are the key characteristics of high technology medicine (Jones *et al.* 1979; Shovelton 1989; Guillemin and Holstrom 1986). For others, such medicine is more a set of beliefs and practices (Cockburn 1988).

A crucial point in all these images is that they appear to be focused where science and medicine meet through the medium of 'high technology'. Indeed the potency of the idea arises precisely because it represents the tangible transformation of science into medicine (Rosenberg 1976). The laboratory becomes the clinic; the workbench becomes the patient; and the experimental scientist becomes the caring doctor rendering the benefits of science through the application of high technology. Whilst some, particularly those clinically engaged in the application of such technologies, may resent what appears to be an over-(melo)dramatic view of their activities, it is not possible to deny the cultural significance of the powerful images which condition everyday understandings of high technology medicine in Britain and the United States.

A panoply of different but related interests are now directly involved in the process of developing and implementing high technologies in clinical practice. Amongst them are clinicians seeking technologies to protect, maintain or improve the health of their patients, and their own professional practices (Koenig 1988); governments seeking to contain overall medical costs, and to reap the political rewards of more sophisticated and modern health care (Banta and Kemp 1982; Stocking 1982); pharmaceutical and other commercial organisations seeking additional opportunities for profit (Gereffi 1983); local managers of medical services seeking more cost effective ways of spending their health care budgets (Jennett 1988b); and scientists developing careers based on the (eventual) clinical applicability of their research in science based medicine (Roch 1980; Wolf and Berle 1980).

Lay attitudes to high technology medicine both reflect and condition the expectations and hopes that are embedded in the promise of science and the power of medicine. In this kind of environment it is not surprising that so many current images of high technology medicine are linked either to the creation of human life, or to the postponement of human death. Yet, at the same time that the application of high technology medicine appears to hold out possibilities for increased longevity and a higher quality of life, these developments are also viewed with underlying suspicion and concern.

Some of these concerns are linked to its perceived capacity to 'dehumanise' medical care, essentially replacing rather than complementing the personal relationships often considered essential to good medicine (Cohen 1993). Others fear the potential for the commercial exploitation of medical care, and the ensuing complete focus of clinical medicine round those aspects of such care which are capable of being 'technologised', which they argue is a process extending to all aspects of medical care (see Roth and Ruzek 1986). Yet others are concerned with the variations in the availability and application of such technologies and their associated costs, as well as their relationship to the ethics of health care (Jennett 1989). The issues of power and control over the development and application of the technologies exercise others (Larkin 1978, 1983), as well as questions concerning their capacity for enhancing or restricting the choices that individuals may be able to make about their lives and health (Kaufert and Locker 1990). At an even broader level there is deep concern about the relationship of the increasing range of technologies to the meaning of life and death, and to our understanding of ourselves and others (Ratcliffe 1989).

UNDERSTANDING LIFE IN THE CONTEXT OF HIGH TECHNOLOGY MEDICINE

C. P. Snow, in reflecting on his earlier Rede Lectures at Cambridge in 1959, focused on molecular biology in 1964 as being not only the epitome of scientific culture, but also the area of scientific research most likely to have a profound social impact. He thereby foresaw the vigorous debates that are now ensuing about the nature and meaning of life, which have been largely contingent on the rapidly accelerating pace of research in the field, as well as contingent on the increasingly bold claims made for the value of this research in relation to human health.

However striking its potential applications might be, when molecular biology appeared to be confined to the experimental laboratory and therefore to take place largely backstage, broader public issues were largely muted. Now however the almost weekly revelation of the precise genetic locii of more and more of the 10,000 or so human diseases currently known to be based on genetic mutations has in itself firmly placed the debates in the public arena, as patient groups, as well as those clinically concerned with the implications of the findings, seek to come to terms with them. In so doing, the issues which these findings raise have begun to receive even broader attention, with the realisation that they may challenge our understanding not only of the causes and management of disease in individuals, but also of the nature of individual identity – who we are, and who we want to be – and the delicate fabric of our relationships with other people.

The initiation of the clinical applications of molecular biology in mass screening programmes, as well as in more long standing but increasingly refined kinds of prenatal testing, has been an important catalyst in the enhanced public profile of this kind of medical intervention (Royal College of Physicians 1989; Weatherall 1991). Moreover, the fusion in the minds of many between such developments, and those associated with reproductive technologies of all kinds has increased the range of those now participating in this discussion (Ratcliffe 1989; Richards 1989; Rothman 1986; Stanworth 1987) . A further dimension has been added with the very beginnings of gene therapy in individuals (Joyce 1990), a prospect which was once thought to be in the distant future.

There have been several immediate concerns for those clinically involved in this substantial and growing area of medical practice – apart from the technical viability and clinical safety of the procedures themselves. Most of these concerns have revolved on the one hand round the financial costs and (perceived medical) benefits of the procedures (Royal College of Physicians 1989; Radcliffe-Richards and Bobrow 1991), and on the other hand round the personal acceptance and response of individuals undergoing, or being offered, them (Green 1990; Green *et al.* 1992; Lippman *et al.* 1985; Marteau 1989). Such concerns are both entirely legitimate and not at all surprising, for clinical care within science based medicine, has always been built on the application of relevant skills and resources to the medically defined problems of individuals.

Nonetheless concerns of a different order which are set in a different context are now being widely debated. On the one hand these concerns are about hard and tangible issues such as who has power over, and control of, both the development, and the use of the new and rapidly increasing number of procedures (Clarke 1991; Lippman 1991; Stacey 1988 Chapter 17). In this respect much concern has been focused on the degree to which those at the receiving end of such clinical interventions, especially women, are generally empowered or disempowered by the availability of the procedures and the ways in which they are applied (Beinart 1990; Cockburn 1988; Stanworth 1987). On the other hand there are less tangible issues arising from these new developments – their effects for example on the broader cultural and social beliefs and practices through which everyday life is managed.

However these two kinds of issues are not separated in practice, for our understanding of our capacity to influence events and circumstances – such as the exercise of personal power and control over such new technologies – is substantially influenced by prevailing cultural beliefs and practices about what is possible and acceptable. Similarly those beliefs and practices are themselves interlocked with, and, in such structures as organised science based medicine, through which key kinds of power and control are mediated and deployed.

Four chapters focus on the profound implications of the clinical applications of molecular genetics for those individuals who are subject to them, and for our general understanding of social and cultural life. Bobrow and Manners, from a position actively engaged in the clinical application of the findings of molecular genetics, note the pace and importance of the new developments. However, whilst acknowledging the range of medical practice to which the developments could relate, they argue that technical and practical factors will circumscribe their application far more than the most vigorous critics will admit. Thus Bobrow and Manners caution against alarmist views of the social consequences of potential clinical applications, but nonetheless state the need for an informed debate leading to a consensus position on such applications.

Richards and Green focus on the complex psychological and social consequences of the rapid increase in prenatal and screening tests, stemming from the findings of molecular biology. For the majority of women who have no prior reason to believe that genetic abnormalities may be detected, the tests appear to slip into the accepted everyday routine of antenatal medical care. Substantially increasing the flow of information to such women is strictly necessary for informed debate, and indeed is necessary for effective individual consent to the tests, yet such information may correspondingly increase levels of anxiety and concern. Richards and Green argue that an open debate on this issue will occur by default or by design, given the speed with which new tests are being introduced, and the rapid widening of their clientele.

Kenen considers the international Human Genome Initiative (HGI). She has grave concerns about what she argues to be the socially ill-informed nature of current scientific research in this area. Kenen believes that large new classes of 'potentially sick' persons will emerge from the development of clinical applications. The social and personal status of such persons found early in life to have a genetic abnormality affecting their (distant) future health or that of their children, may be extremely damaged. In addition the range of potential clinical applications arising from the research on the HGI is likely to have profound general social consequences.

Strathern considers the relationship of the new reproductive technologies to current ideas about kinship. She argues that the technologies are not just technical procedures, but that they are associated with forms of knowledge about kinship – in particular about the nature of who we are in relation to 'our kin'. The new technologies have allowed the possibility of the separation of procreation from reproduction, and therefore the possibility of separating individual (genetic) identity from a relationship with another which has hitherto formed the common Euro-American understanding of what 'kinship' is. Strathern then reflects on the displacement effects of knowledge related to new reproductive technologies.

SOCIAL AND ETHICAL ISSUES IN MANAGING HIGH TECHNOLOGY MEDICINE

As the clinical applications of molecular biology have begun to open up serious questions about the meaning of life in relation to its beginning, the application of other technologies has focused attention on the maintenance of human life which may be nearing its end. The development of advanced surgical techniques assisted by an array of associated technologies – including machinery to replace certain body functions in the short or medium term, or the use of transplanted organs or tissues from human donors – has focused attention on the circumstances in which such technologies should be deployed (Jennett 1986).

The powerful objective of saving life, as much embedded in everyday lay aims as it is formally part of the expectations and commitments of formal medical care, has traditionally tended to overwhelm critical questions about the means by which this objective is achieved, and the consequences of the process. However as it is increasingly possible to save, and thereafter to maintain 'life' in many forms through the use of various technological interventions, the quality of that life and its personal, social and ethical standing has been subject to considerable scrutiny (Jennett 1991). Intense debate has been continuing, particularly in relation to the boundary between life and death, and as to how such a boundary can be medically (re-)established, be widely accepted and be presented to give clear options for clinicians, patients and their relatives (JAMA 1968; President's Commission 1983; Stanley 1989). Difficult and celebrated cases (most notably that of Quinlan in the United States (Quinlan *et al.* 1977)) have pointed up the complex issues, and have crystallised the need for further and explicit guidelines about such situations. Nonetheless, the ethical and practical basis of such guidelines do not remain unchallenged (Cohen 1993), as different cases and different issues arising out of the life saving role of high technology medicine present further dilemmas. The debate about these dilemmas has now focused on the relationship between the relative costs and benefits of the procedures and how they might be measured (Jennett 1988a; Jennett 1990), and their association with relevant ethical considerations (Cubbon 1991; Jennett 1987). Whilst some argue that there is an effective fusion between economic and ethical criteria for judging the benefits of high technology medicine (Williams 1992), others suggest that this view fails to acknowledge a range of other important factors which cannot be incorporated within an economic evaluation of the technology concerned (Ashmore et al. 1989; Harris 1987; Smith 1987).

Further issues associated with the use of life saving technologies relate to the consequences for those who might be considered crucial third parties to their application. For example, the use of body organs or tissues of others has often become an important feature of such technologies (Plough 1986). The means by which such organs and tissues are obtained, who they are obtained from, and what interests the donor (alive or dead) and the 'harvester' of the organs and tissues have in their future use, raise a series of questions which tap the intellectual margins of legal and ethical knowledge (Rettig 1989). These issues are additionally complicated by the involvement of commercial interests in the management of this process, and their development of further products from the original source of organs and tissues.

Four chapters address important debates concerning the development, use and evaluation of life saving technologies, and particularly address the role of commercial exploitation of high technology products in relation to medical practice. Jennett's main concern is the relationship between the ethical and economic aspects of high technology medicine, particularly in so far as it relates to surgery in life threatening situations. He indicates that there is no necessary conflict between the economic and ethical status of decisions about when such technologies should be used, indeed the two are inextricably interlinked. Thus Jennett argues for a concerted and systematic approach to evaluating the costs and benefits of the technologies.

Preston documents the problems in developing new technology, with a case study of the recent history of the development and use of the artificial heart in the United States. He indicates that there are salutary lessons to be learnt from the premature and highly public application of this technology. In particular the combination of commercial pressures and ambitious clinicians has led to a speculative and contentious technology being therapeutically employed before it had been fully researched, and without its social implications being considered. Preston draws the conclusion that social and political control over the development and dissemination of new technologies is essential.

Following Preston's analysis of commercial pressures in relation to one new technology, Freeman focuses on legal debates which are now resulting from the commercial exploitation of body products. In particular he analyses the case of *Moore* v *Regents of the University of California* in which the ownership of profitable cell lines developed from a patient was debated. The key question was whether the patient (Moore) had property rights in his own body products. The court concluded that under existing law he did not, and Freeman argues that the court's conclusion and its reasoning is defective, and does not meet the complex challenge posed by developments in biotechnology.

Erin and Harris take Freeman's argument further and discuss and elaborate what they believe could be an ethically sound system of commerce in body products, given a general presumption that trade in such products could be countenanced. They address ethical objections that could be levied against such a system, and conclude that what they call a 'monopsonistic market' – that is a market where one buyer exists for a range of sellers – would provide the most satisfactory system, with a series of additional ethical safeguards.

THE CULTURAL CONTEXT OF CHOICE IN RELATION TO HIGH TECHNOLOGY MEDICINE

Most developments in high technology medicine can be argued to be based on (or to assume) some common set of cultural expectations, shared by those involved in giving and receiving medical care. These expectations are not only about, for example, the goal of saving life, but also relate to the style, manner and means by which that goal is accomplished, and indeed the circumstances in which the goal may be considered inappropriate.

In this respect, as was noted earlier, criticisms are sometimes levied against forms of high technology medicine for what may be described as their actually, or potentially, 'dehumanising' qualities (Ratcliffe 1989). This criticism not only relates to the technology itself constituting a physical, as well as a personal and social barrier between doctor and patient, but is also based on the idea that there is a clinical momentum which is contained in the very use of the technology, which is not controlled, nor is controllable by a human – doctor's – hand (Angell 1990). The fear is of a technological imperative in medical care in which the means to specified (human) ends become subverted by those means which become ends in themselves (Koenig 1988; Wolf and Berle 1980). The issue is thus not only that technologies as objects cannot be considered as possessing the capacity to be caring or sensitive to human needs, but that decisions about the outcomes of technological involvement are embedded in the technology itself.

Of course the counter argument to this position is that clinical medicine may use high technology as a resource, but it is only one amongst a number of more traditional resources all firmly within the doctors's clinical control. Indeed such a resource may allow far more informed choices, for both doctor and patient, through enhanced diagnostic or treatment possibilities, than those which would be available without the technology (Jennett 1992). Moreover there is no reason to believe that the doctor in this situation is likely to be more, or less 'insensitive' or 'uncaring' than in any other clinical setting.

Exploring this issue of sensitivity to the needs of individuals in a broader context, the cultural meanings of serious illness, and of death and dying must be considered as just as important as medical judgements about when death is considered to have occurred. Indeed medical, as much as any other understandings of when death happens are themselves based on specific (biomedical) cultural beliefs and practices. Such an observation is particularly important in discussing possible conflicts of interpretation and meaning in the use of high technology medicine at this very significant time (Campbell and Campbell 1978; Jones *et al.* 1979; Shovelton 1989). Many everyday (lay) understandings of the meaning of life threatening illness, and how it should be treated may not be similar to, let alone identical with, those of clinicians (Wilson-Barnett 1979). However the latter may make strenuous attempts within their own framework to come to terms with those lay definitions – to consult and attempt to agree procedures and outcomes with patients and their relatives. But such a resolution of the situation is particularly complex in relation to cultural differences between doctors and their patients, who may only partially share the doctor's beliefs about the meaning of life, and the place of life threatening illness within it (Fox and Swazey 1978; Strauss *et al.* 1985). Such problems are becoming more common as communities with different ethnic identities – and often based on different systems of religious practices and beliefs – come into contact with high technology medicine in life threatening situations (Lock and Gordon 1988). The global mobility of clinicians trained in science based medicine, and the ubiquity of such medicine as part of the health care system of almost every society (Banta and Kemp 1982), may mean that these kinds of problems are likely to occur with even greater frequency. In this setting the basis of, and the opportunities for, choices in relation to health – for the individuals involved, as well as for the communities of which they are a part – deserve special attention.

Three chapters address questions related to the context of choice in medical care. Higgs starts from the perspective that relatively recent medical developments – including more accurate diagnosis as well as enhanced therapeutic options – have given both patients and medical staff more options at points close to death. The role of high technology medicine in relation to these developments is ambiguous – it may increase some options, but runs the risk of being inappropriately used. Higgs also argues that certain features of dying cannot be handled by technological interventions, and must be dealt with sensitively with respect for the wishes and the individual identity of the person concerned.

Lock places the analysis of Higgs in a cross-cultural context by noting the power and resilience of traditional beliefs towards the management of death in Japan. Such beliefs and associated practices are shown up most sharply in continuing controversies about the possibility of heart transplantation in Japan. Lock documents the nature of these controversies and conflicts, and argues that there may be important lessons to be learned in the West from the style, as well as the content of these debates.

Frankenberg argues that fundamental cultural differences underlie the ways in which doctors and patients approach, and understand surgical treatments for heart disease. Working through the idea of 'embodied knowledge' Frankenberg demonstrates how the understanding of bodily experiences at, or about, the times in which 'crises of the heart' occur reflect cultural differences in the interpretation of these phenomena. Using descriptions of heart conditions in medical and nursing texts as well as novels, Frankenberg explores their meaning and relationship to each other in the practice of medicine.

UNDERSTANDING THE SOCIAL ROLE AND DEVELOPMENT OF HIGH TECHNOLOGY MEDICINE

The extent to which technologies have now become a routine component of most medical care is a theme which is taken up by certain analysts. Science based medicine is conceived of as dependent on an increasing array of technologies which shaped by processes – some would say forces – related to its professional structure and organisation have come to dominate increasingly broad fields of health care. In part the issue which this argument poses is a definitional one. Early in this account Banta's definition of technologies (1983) was used to begin the analysis. His view of what constituted technologies was a broad one embracing drugs, devices, medical and surgical procedures, together with their support and organisational structures. Using such a perspective it would be hard to conclude that almost any aspect of contemporary medical care was not based on, or employed, significant technologies.

However this definition can be taken even further by arguing that there is what might be described as a 'technological way' of undertaking medicine through a combination of sets of beliefs and practices which redefine or create new areas of application. In this framework it becomes possible to consider technologies, or even 'high technologies', as processes and practices, rather than entities. Of particular importance to this line of argument are analyses derived from the work of Foucault (1973) and their emphasis on, for example, 'technologies of the self'. In this respect the human sciences have become the new technologies, and human scientists have become the new technologists of medicine (Arney and Bergen 1984; Rose 1990). Through developing techniques and instruments to measure the psychosocial aspects of emerging and broader medical concerns, a new battery of sophisticated technologies is being added by human scientists to the array of those that currently exist. This development in itself can also be considered to constitute an explicit critique of the more traditional kinds of high technology medicine, as the psychosocial domain of health care assumes greater and greater importance.

Such an approach is not the only way in which the social context of high technology medicine can be explored. Other approaches emphasise the role of everyday knowledge about medical technologies not just as an abstract set of ideas, nor as a set of objects and procedures met whilst a patient is under medical care, but as deeply embedded in our understanding of ourselves, and our personal and social life. Such technologies may be used as a basis of defining what is an appropriate and 'natural' way of managing health crises, and indeed as a way of defining the boundaries beyond which technologically based medicine should not be involved. Further, drawing on discussions earlier in this account, the construction of personhood – of personal identity – is in many ways bound up with particular images and practices of high technology medicine, which fuse with general concerns about the fears and hopes of science, and scientific endeavour.

Four chapters focus on ways in high technology medicine has become part of the social worlds of more and more people, either directly through the extension of the domain of medical concerns, or through the existence of knowledge and practices related to such medicine. Calnan and Williams ground their discussion of the lay understanding of scientific medicine in a recent social survey in Britain. They demonstrate that there is a generally positive attitude towards most technologies employed in modern scientific medicine, whether they be surgical procedures, drugs, or other technologies. However underlying this broadly positive view are concerns about some features of scientific medicine. Calnan and Williams thus develop a typology of lay evaluations as a template against which particular technologies can be considered in lay terms to tend towards either being 'good' or 'bad'.

Armstrong, in taking a different but complementary direction to Calnan and Williams, focuses on the ways in which historical developments in technologies have come to constitute and reflect medicine itself, as well as those subject to it including medical practitioners and 'the patient'. Developing the arguments of Foucault he demonstrates how the 'psychosocial' space of the patient has come to be a key area in which modern medicine is practised. This development is also reflected in the increasing role of 'human scientists' in analysing medical endeavours, including the concerted examination of social consequences of high technology medicine itself.

In considering the rapid growth of medical rehabilitation Robinson echoes Armstrong in pointing to the extent to which psychological and social issues have come to play a larger and larger part in the rehabilitation process. Nonetheless the use of high technologies in, for example, attempts to dramatically alter the consequences of spinal cord injury, and to manage other severe and long term bodily damage, has raised many issues about the role of such technologies, and their social and cultural consequences.

Lyon's analysis is of the development of modern medicine into further areas of human life, particular those which seek to relate 'the body' and 'the mind' together through the new field of psychoneuroimmunology. Lyon argues, in her review, that a way of integrating these new approaches, and their implicit emphasis on both neurophysical and social life, is through the 'bridge' of emotion.

CONCLUSION

This analysis takes the arguments about the role of high technology medicine through and beyond individual cases, to discuss its broader social and cultural consequences. Such medicine – however it is defined – might be considered as just representing a modest extension of an already wide range of existing medical practices, and thereby not raising radically new issues, dilemmas or concerns. However the following accounts indicate that, at the very least, practices in and around high technology medicine have sharpened many social, cultural, ethical and economic debates. These debates as well as high technology medicine itself are at the cutting edge of life and death.

REFERENCES

Angell, M. (1990), 'Prisoners of technology: the case of Nancy Cruzan', *New England Journal of Medicine*, CCCXXII, pp. 1226–8

Arney, W. and Bergen, B. (1984), *Medicine and the Management of Living*, Chicago University Press

Ashmore, M., Mulkay, M. and Pinch, T. (1989), *Health and Efficiency: A Sociology of Health Economics*, Open University Press, Milton Keynes

Banta, H.D. (1983), 'Social science research on medical technology: utility and limitations' *Social Science and Medicine*, XVII, pp. 1363–9

Banta, H. D. and Kemp, K. B. (eds.) (1982) *The Management of Health Care Technology in Nine Countries*, Springer Publishing Company, New York

Barley, S. R. (1988), 'The social construction of a machine: ritual, superstition, magical thinking and other pragmatic responses to running a CT scanner', in M. Lock, D. Gordon, (eds.), *Biomedicine Examined*, Kluwer Academic Publishers, Dordrecht

Beinart, J. (1990), 'Obstetric analgesia and the control of childbirth in twentieth-century Britain', in J. Garcia, R. Fitzpatrick, N. Richards, (eds.), *The Politics of Maternity Care*, Clarendon Press, Oxford

Bell, S. E. (1989) 'Technology in medicine: development, diffusion and health policy', in H. E. Freman and S. Levine (eds.), *Handbook of Medical Sociology*, 4th edn, Prentice Hall, Englewood Cliffs, pp. 185–204

Bijker, W. E., Hughes, T. P. and Pinch, T. J. (eds.), *The Social Construction of Technological*

Systems: New Directions in the Sociology and History of Technology, MIT Press, Cambridge, Mass.

Campbell, J. D. and Campbell, A. R. (1978), 'The social and economic costs of end-stage renal disease: a patient's perspective', *New England Journal of Medicine,* CCIC, pp. 386–92

Clarke, A. (1991) 'Is non-directive genetic counselling possible?', *The Lancet,* CCCXXXVIII, pp. 998–1001

Cockburn, C. (1988), *Machinery of Dominance: Women, Men and Technical Know-how,* Northeastern University Press, Boston

Cohen, S. (1993), *Whose Life is it Anyhow?,* Robson Books, London

Cubbon, J. (1991), 'The principle of QALY maximisation as the basis for allocating health care resources', *Journal of Medical Ethics,* XVII, pp. 181–4

Davis, A.B. (1978), 'Medical technology', in T. I. Williams, *A History of Technology,* Clarendon Press, Oxford, vol. 7, pp. 1316–62

Dominguez, E. A., Bar-Sela, A.and Musher, D. M. (1987), 'Adoption of thermometry into clinical practice in the United States', *Reviews of Infectious Diseases,* IX, pp. 1193–201

Foote, S.B. (1987), 'Assessing medical technology assessment: past, present and future', *Milbank Quarterly,* LXV, pp. 59–80

Foucault, M. (1973), *The Birth of the Clinic: An Archaeology of Medical Perception,* Tavistock, London

Fox R. C. and Swazey, J. P. (1978), *The Courage to Fail: A Social View of Organ Transplants and Dialysis,* 2nd edn, University of Chicago Press

Gabe, J. and Calnan, M. (1989), 'The limits of medicine: women's perception of medical technology', *Social Science and Medicine,* XXVIII, pp. 223–31

Gereffi, G. (1983), *The Pharmaceutical Industry and Dependency in the Third World,* Princeton University Press

Green, J. M., Statham, H. and Snowdon, C. (1992), 'Screening for fetal abnormality: attitudes and experiences', in T. Chard, M. P. M. Richards, (eds.), *Obstetrics in the 1990s: Current Controversies,* Clinics in Developmental Medicine 123/124, Mac Keith Press, London

Green, J. M. (1990), *Calming or Harming: A Critical Review of Psychological Effects of Fetal Diagnosis on Pregnant Women,* Galton Institute Occasional Papers, Second Series No. 2, London

Guillemin, J. and Holstrom, L.L. (1986), *Mixed Blessings: Intensive Care for Newborns,* Oxford University Press

Harris, J. (1991), 'Unprincipled QALYs: a response to Cubbon', *Journal of Medical Ethics,* XVII, pp. 185–8

Harris, J. (1987), 'Qualifying the value of life', *Journal of Medical Ethics,* XIII, pp. 117–23

Institute of Medicine, (1985), *Assessing Medical Technologies,* Committee for Evaluating Medical Technologies in Clinical Use, National Academy Press, Washington, DC

JAMA (1968), 'A Definition of Irreversible Coma: Report of the Harvard Medical School to Examine the Definition of Brain Death', *Journal of the American Medical Association,* CCV, pp. 337–40

Jennett, B. (1986), *High Technology Medicine: Benefits and Burdens,* Oxford University Press

—— (1987) 'Are ethics and economics incompatible in health care?', *Proceedings of the Royal College of Physicians of Edinburgh*, XVII, pp. 190–5

—— (1988a) 'Balancing benefits and burdens of surgery', *British Medical Bulletin*, XLIV, pp. 499–513

—— (1988b) 'HTM and the elderly', in M. Wells, C. Freer (eds.), *Health Problems of an Ageing Population*, Macmillan, London, pp. 177–90

—— (1988c), 'Assessment of clinical technologies: importance for provision and use', *International Journal of Technology Assessment in Health Care*, IV, pp. 435–45

—— (1989), 'Quality of care and cost containment in the US and UK', *Theoretical Medicine*, X, pp. 207–15

—— (1990), 'Is intensive care worthwhile?', *Care of the Critical Illness*, III, pp. 85–8

—— (1991), 'Decisions to limit the use of technologies that save or sustain life', *Proceedings of the Royal College of Physicians of Edinburgh*, XX, pp. 407–15

Jones, J., Hoggart, B., Withey, J., Donaghue, K. and Ellis, B.W. (1979), 'What the patients say: a study of reactions to an intensive care unit', *Intensive Care Medicine*,V, pp. 89–92

Joyce, C. (1990), 'Four-year-old is first gene therapy patient', *New Scientist*, 22 September 1990, p. 25

Katz, J. (ed.) (1972), *Experimentation with Human Beings*, Russell Sage Foundation, New York

Kaufert, J. M. and Locker, D. (1990), 'Rehabilitation ideology and respiratory support technology', *Social Science and Medicine*, XXX, pp. 867–77

Koenig, B. A. (1988), 'The technological imperative in medical practice: social creation of a "routine" treatment', in M. Lock. and D. Gordon, (eds.), *Biomedicine Examined*, Kluwer Academic Publishers, Dordrecht

Larkin, G. V. (1978), 'Medical dominance and control: radiographers in the division of labour', *Sociological Review*, XXVI, pp. 843–58

—— (1983), *Occupational Monopoly and Modern Medicine*, Tavistock Publications, London

Lippman, A. (1991), 'Prenatal genetic testing and screening: cnstructing needs and reinforcing inequalities', *American Journal of Law and Medicine*, XVII, pp. 15–50

Lippman, A., Perry, T. B., Mandel, S. an d Cartier, S. (1985), 'Chorionic villi sampling: women's attitudes', *American Journal of Medical Genetics*, XXII, pp. 395–401

Lock, M. and Gordon, D. (1988), *Biomedicine Examined*, Kluwer Academic Publishing, Dordrecht

Marteau, T. M. (1989), 'Psychological costs of screening', *British Medical Journal*, CCLXLIX, p. 527

Plough, A. L. (1986), *Borrowed Time: Artificial Organs and the Politics of Extending Lives*, Temple University Press, Philadephia

President's Commission for the Study of Ethical Problems in Medicine and Biomedical and Behavioral Research (1983), *Deciding to Forego Life Sustaining Treatment: Ethical and Legal Issues in Treatment Decisions*, US Government Printing Office, Washington, D.C.

Quill, T. E. (1991), 'Death and dignity: a case of individual decision-making', *New England Journal of Medicine*, CCCXXIV, p. 691

Quinlan, J. and Quinlan, J., with Battelle, P. (1977), *Karen Ann: The Quinlans Tell Their Story*, Doubleday Anchor, New York

Radcliffe-Richards, J. and Bobrow, M. (1991), 'Ethical issues in clinical genetics', *Journal of the Royal College of Physicians*, XXV

Ratcliffe, K.S. (1989), *Healing Technology: Feminist Perspectives*, University of Michigan Press, Ann Arbor

Reiser, S. (1978), *Medicine and the Reign of Technology*, Cambridge University Press

Rettig, R. A. (1989), 'The politics of organ transplantation: a parable of our time', *Journal of Health Politics, Policy and Law*, XIV, pp. 191–227

Richards, M. P. M. (1989), 'Social and ethical problems of fetal diagnosis and screening'. *Journal of Reproductive and Infant Psychology*, VII, pp. 171–85

Roch, E. B. (1980), 'Process of innovation in medical technology: American research on ultrasound. 1947 to 1962', Ph.D thesis, University of Pennsylvania

Rose, N. (1990), *Governing the Soul*, Routledge, London

Rosenberg, C. (1976), 'Martin Arrowsmith: the scientist as hero', in C. Rosenberg, *No Other Gods: On Science and American Social Thought*, Johns Hopkins University Press, Baltimore, pp. 123–31

Roth, J. A. and Ruzek, S. B. (eds.) (1986), *The Adoption and Social Consequences of Medical Technologies*, Research in the Sociology of Health Care, vol. 4, JAI Press, Greenwich

Rothman, B. K. (1986), *The Tentative Pregnancy*, Viking, New York

Royal College of Physicians (1989), *Prenatal Diagnosis and Genetic Screening: Community and Service Implications*, Royal College of Physicians, London

Rublee, D. A. (1989), 'Medical technology in Canada, Germany and the United States', *Health Affairs*, XIX, pp. 178–81

Scott, W. R. (1990), 'Innovation in medical care organizations: a synthetic review', *Medical Care Review*, XLVII, pp. 165–92

Shovelton, D. S. (1989), 'Reflections on an intensive therapy unit', *British Medical Journal*, I, pp. 737–8

Smith, A. (1987), 'Qualms about QALYs', *Lancet*, II, pp. 1134–6

Snow, C. P. (1964), *The Two Cultures: A Second Look*, Cambridge University Press

Stacey, M. (1988), *The Sociology of Health and Healing*, Unwin Hyman, London

Stanley, J. M. (1989), 'The Appleton consensus: suggested international guidelines for decisions to forgo life- prolonging medical treatment', *Journal of Medical Ethics*, XV, pp. 129–36

Stanworth, M. (ed.), (1987), *Reproductive Technologies: Gender, Motherhood and Medicine*, University of Minnesota Press, Minn.

Stocking, B. (1982), 'The management of medical technology in the United Kingdom', in H. D. Banta, K. B. Kemp, *The Management of Health Care Technology in Nine Countries*, Springer Publishing Company, New York, pp. 10–27

Strauss, A., Fagerhaugh, S., Suczek, B. and Wiener, C. (1985), *Social Organization of Medical Work*, University of Chicago Press

Weatherall, D. J. (1991), *The New Genetics and Clinical Practice*, 3rd edn, Oxford University Press

Williams, A. (1992), 'Cost effective analysis: is it ethical?', *Journal of Medical Ethics*, XVIII, pp. 7–11

Wilson-Barnett, J. (1979), 'A review of research into the experience of patients suffering from coronary thrombosis', *International Journal of Nursing Studies*, XVI, pp. 185–87

Wolf, S. and Berle, B. B. (1980), *The Technological Imperative in Medicine*, Plenum Press, New York

PART ONE

Understanding life in the context of high technology medicine

2

The social consequencs of advances in the clinical applications of genetics

MARTIN BOBROW AND ELIZABETH MANNERS

INTRODUCTION

The advent of molecular genetic techniques in the 1980s initiated a revolution in biological research as far-reaching as any since it was first learned that organisms are composed of cells. Predictably, such new insights bring opportunities for both good and harm. The ethical aspects of human genetics have been much discussed recently (*Nature* 1991b). That such attention has been paid to these issues is particularly due to continuing awareness of the influence of eugenics on political actions in Europe in the 1930s and 1940s. It is also because of the very high media profile achieved by the grandiose 'Human Genome Project', whose objective is to determine the entire sequence of the human genetic complement, and which has therefore been portrayed as the ultimate feature of biological reductionism.

Genetics is about inheritance, and the cellular control of embryological development. It is thus distinct from the study of fertilization and early pregnancy. New techniques of artificial fertilization, although they clinically interact with the genetic means of determining the potential characteristics of a pre-implantation embryo, are not in themselves 'Genetics'. In its clinical applications, genetics focuses on prediction based on the uniformity of the genome in all normal cells of an individual. As all the cells of an individual's body (with minor exceptions) normally carry the same gene complement, and because these genes will eventually exert their effect on that individual, it is possible to sample any organ or tissue, at any developmental stage, and to learn what is likely to befall different tissues at different times.

Thus it is possible to remove a sample of the placenta at 10 weeks gestation, and to learn of the virtually inevitable onset of a degenerative disorder of the nervous system that will not become clinically manifest until 40 or 50 years after birth (Royal College of Physicians 1989; Brock *et al.* 1990; Skraastad *et al.* 1991). This power of prediction appears awesome, but is limited, because the probability of the prediction being accurate depends on the extent to which the characteristic in question is under purely genetic control independent of environmental modification. For several thousand relatively uncommon disorders, such as Huntington's chorea (the progressive degenerative disease of the nervous system alluded to above), muscular dystrophy, and cystic fibrosis, environmental modification of genetic effects is indeed minimal, and the accuracy of prediction is correspondingly very high. However, in some of the more common diseases of adult life – e.g. diabetes, coronary artery disease, or schizophrenia – the situation is more problematic. Although familial aggregation of the conditions suggests an important genetic contribution, they do not follow the simple rules of inheritance which characterize disorders due to the effect of single genes. There are two sources of variation, and their implications are fundamentally different from one another.

First, there are the effects of other genes: which is to say that some disorders result not from an overwhelming defect in one genetic function, but from a more subtle interplay between the effects of two or more genes. Precise illustrations of such disorders are difficult to give at present, but the phenomenon is likely to exist. In principle, as more is learnt of genes and their functions, it will be possible to learn how to analyse and predict the effects of other genes as well. Thus although the research will be more difficult, there is no reason to believe that these so-called 'polygenic traits' will remain forever beyond the reach of genetic prediction.

Second, the more significant source of variation is the interplay between genetic endowment (either simple or complex) and environmental factors, which probably occurs in many common disorders, such as coronary heart disease, diabetes, some malignancies, manic-depressive disorders and schizophrenia (Royal College of Physicians 1989). This important interplay is less amenable to simple prediction. Environmental influences may already be subject to some kinds of intervention when individuals wish to influence their destiny, but even purely genetic conditions will increasingly become amenable to various forms of treatment, and it is wrong to think of genetic disease as necessarily beyond therapeutic ingenuity.

What sorts of procedures are already in place, or are likely to become practically possible over the next 10 – 15 years, which may have significant social consequences? The prenatal diagnosis of inherited disorders has been increasingly practised for some years now. Widescale population screening for 'carriers' of genetic disorders is becoming practicable for some common conditions. Predicting liability to the development of more complex and common adult disorders is in its infancy, but has clearly been initiated. The first faltering steps have been taken towards the development of effective gene therapy. All these developments have both substantial ethical and social implications.

PRENATAL DIAGNOSIS

Samples can be taken either by amniocentesis (usually at about 16 weeks of pregnancy), or by chorion villus (placenta) sampling (at about 10–11 weeks) (Royal College of Physicians 1989). In the future preimplantation diagnosis (within the first week of pregnancy) will probably become possible (Monk 1991). These techniques have allowed hundreds of thousands of couples at risk of serious and currently untreatable genetic disorders to test their pregnancies. The vast majority of tested pregnancies are in fact found to be normal, and the testing procedure therefore provides reassurance rather than increased anxiety, but a minority of cases will show an abnormality. However, a substantial number of families who had previously chosen to remain childless have been prepared to undertake pregnancies because it has become possible to carry out prenatal diagnosis. For instance, Modell et al. (1984) reported that British Cypriot families at risk for thalassaemia major had previously virtually ceased reproduction after an affected child was diagnosed, and sought termination of 70 per cent of all pregnancies. Following the introduction of prenatal diagnosis in 1975, however, nearly normal reproduction was resumed by at-risk families. It seems likely that a substantial part of the population regards prenatal diagnosis as a useful option, although this is a matter for individual choice rather than professional prescription. Issues which have been raised with regard to prenatal diagnosis include:

1. Those related to abortion itself (which is emphatically not a genetic issue).
2. Whether the termination of abnormal pregnancies implies a devalu-

ation of disabled people in general, and, if so, whether it is therefore likely to lead to reduced care and attention for those who need it.

3. Whether economic pressures will be brought to bear by the state or health insurers to avoid abnormal births, even when parents are themselves not persuaded that this is the course of action they wish to follow. In this respect there already exist anecdotal accounts of health insurers refusing cover for future medical expenses where parents have refused prenatal testing and termination.

4. The 'slippery slope' problem of how to control the extension of prenatal diagnosis to less and less serious disorders. In some countries, termination of female pregnancies on purely social grounds has been considered a modern equivalent of infanticide, and has attracted widespread international criticism (Jayaraman 1991). Even without outside pressures, the mere availability of a variety of procedures which improve the likelihood of a normal outcome to pregnancy creates in everyone an expectation of perfection which is quite removed from the natural state of our species, and this may encourage many people to be less accepting of both the risk and the fact of abnormality when it does occur.

None of these issues create intrinsically acute problems in themselves, but they all require a degree of social consensus on the latitude in decision-making that individual parents, and individual health professionals, should have (Royal College of Physicians 1989). A completely libertarian approach to individual choice could lead to the taking of extreme positions by a minority, and possibly to a shift of the centre of opinion, which currently endorses the restricted use of testing and termination for severe and untreatable disorders, into more contentious areas. For example, already one of the authors (MB) has been asked to arrange for testing, with a view to subsequent termination, of a foetus which although healthy, might have been a carrier of a defective gene for a serious disease which would thus have been passed on to a subsequent generation – thus practising a form of intrafamilial eugenics.

However currently prenatal testing is very largely restricted to conditions such as Down's syndrome, cystic fibrosis, and muscular dystrophy, but it is technically already possible to test for a wide variety of other disorders, ranging from known fatal conditions through disorders such as phenylketonuria (which can cause severe mental handicap, but where careful dietary management can control most manifestations), to relatively minor conditions such as colour-blindness. Encouragingly, the availability of prenatal tests does not always create a public demand for their use. Adult onset polycystic kidney disease (which causes renal failure in a high proportion of sufferers) is inherited in a simple way, and prenatal testing has been possible for some years, but there has been virtually no demand for the test itself (Hodgkinson *et al.* 1990). Thus so far it appears that there is little evidence of what might be described as abuse of these tests – through their use for what could be regarded as socially improper ends – suggesting that both public and professional attitudes may be more robust than some have feared.

POPULATION SCREENING

Most couples are only discovered to be at high risk of having a child with a severe genetic abnormality after their first affected child has been born. Shifting the point of diagnosis to a more useful time is the prime objective of population screening – the testing of healthy individuals for abnormal genes which they may be carrying, which could result in the birth of an affected child. In the great majority of genetic disorders, these 'carriers' are themselves healthy, and specific tests are the only means of discovering their genetic status prior to the birth of an affected child.

The principles of carrier screening have been well established in population groups with an unusually high incidence of particular genetic conditions. Thalassaemia in the population of some parts of Italy and Cyprus; sickle cell disease in those of African extraction; and Tay-Sachs disease in Ashkenazi Jews are major examples of well developed and active population screening programmes. These are all disorders which allow carrier detection on the basis of a haematological or biochemical test, rather than through direct gene analysis, and all the programmes were initiated long before the age of molecular genetics. Some thalassaemia programmes have had a marked effect in reducing the birth incidence of what most regard as a very distressing disorder (World Health Organization 1983; Angastiniotis 1990). Intensive Tay-Sachs carrier testing in the USA, Israel and some other countries has also apparently reduced the disease incidence significantly (Kaback 1981). In both these cases, the emphasis has been strongly on community information and education, and achieving the support of community leaders, in order to provide the community with the information that was wanted, in a way that they understood. Sickle cell disease screening in America has had a less happy beginning, and was initially seen as an imposed programme with racial overtones – a perception that was reinforced when some carriers found themselves subject to discrimination in relation to employment (Rutkow and Lipton 1974; Goodman 1989).

The subject of population screening has now been brought to the top of the clinical geneticists' agenda by the cloning of the gene responsible for cystic fibrosis (Riordan *et al.* 1989). It is a disease carried by one in every 25 Europeans. It transpires that the disorder can be caused by a substantial number of different alterations in the gene. Thus at present no single test can detect all cystic fibrosis-causing mutations. The tests that have been devised locate about 85 per cent of carriers (Ng *et al.* 1991). A more important factor than the probable accuracy of the relevant tests, however, is the perception amongst those professionally involved that widespread population screening at this stage would be allowing scientific knowledge to pre-empt necessary understanding of the psychosocial effects of such screening (Marteau 1989, 1990). Arguably carriers detected through such a programme would not obtain any direct and immediate benefit to their health. The results of testing would be to provide information for potential future decisions, in particular the knowledge that if two carriers have children, there is a 25 per cent chance that each child will have the disease. A number of questions are posed by such testing.

Do people who have never previously heard of the condition, or who may not have begun to think of reproduction, or who may not have a long-term partner, want such information? What is the best age at which to conduct such testing? Testing during pregnancy itself is organizationally very convenient, but the options available to those tested at 18 weeks are very limited compared to those tested at an earlier stage. However it is not clear how information given as a result of testing will be understood. Will the information be remembered, and the range of possible and appropriate actions be taken (Zeesman *et al.* 1984)? Or is it possible that in many years time individuals will be encountered who have misunderstood the implications of a normal test result and have thus resolved to live a childless life? Examples from mass cancer screening programmes suggest the possibility of such misunderstandings.

Comprehending the results of genetic tests, and the associated probabilistic information on the health of future offspring, has been shown to be difficult for those previously unacquainted with such ideas (Frets *et al.* 1991). Clinical geneticists convey such information in the process of genetic counselling; however this process involves lengthy and intensive face-to-face sessions with a highly trained professional counsellor. Such a practice cannot be deployed if several million adults are subject to screening. There are a variety of views (Beaudet 1990; Caskey *et al.* 1990; *Lancet* 1990)on how information on the results of genetic tests may be given, but there is no clear research evidence as to which approach is the most effective. There is a lack of knowledge as to how to convey information, how effective it will be, and whether a highly organized programme of information giving would be generally beneficial. Finally there is little clear evidence as to the general public demand for, or interest in, such information.

Estimates of the uptake rates for population screening, when it has been offered in a few pilot projects (Williamson *et al.* 1991; Ten Kate and Tjimstra 1989; Kaplan *et al.* 1991) varied from 10 per cent to 80 per cent. It is possible that the uptake rates depended as much on the energy and enthusiasm put into the recruiting process, as on any other factor. Advertising their services may thus be just as crucial for geneticists as for other service providers. However one issue which arises from such an active recruitment process is whether enthusiastic sponsorship of a screening programme by those altruistically involved may amount to a form of coercion. Such an issue requires public debate rather than professional judgement alone, especially in countries where screening programmes may be commercially sponsored.

The potentially problematic side-effects of such programmes may be unresolved anxiety, the social stigmatization of carriers, and a possible failure to understand the information provided. Such difficulties may be compounded by genuine scientific errors in the test process. There are sound grounds, and some firm evidence, for believing that all of these adverse outcomes will occur. Thus the resolution of these issues is important before large scale screening is implemented.

So far, the discussion has been concerned with potential parents and the health of their potential offspring, but there are of course other situations where genetic tests can predict disorders which will affect the health of the individual being tested. These 'predictive' or 'presymptomatic' tests apply in dominantly inherited disorders such as polycystic kidney disease and Huntington's chorea (Huggins *et al.* 1990; Journal of Medical Genetics 1990). The presence of an abnormal gene predicts the onset of a disorder many years before its clinical symptoms become manifest. There is a considerable (although still inconclusive) body of literature concerning the problems of predictive testing in 'high-risk' situations – for example, in the relatives of affected people, who are themselves at significant risk of having inherited the abnormal gene. In conditions such as familial adenomatous polyposis, which leads to colon cancer, the rationale for testing is strong, because arly warning allows clinical screening programmes to be implemented which will be of direct benefit to the patient. However where a genetic test provides information but no immediate possibility of therapy, it may facilitate lifestyle and reproductive planning, but will not enable the onset or course of the disease to be altered. The technical possibility of mass population screening for disorders of this type has not yet presented itself, and there has been little attention paid to its possible consequences.

POPULATION SCREENING AND INSURANCE

A particularly important context in which general large scale public health screening already takes place is in relation to health insurance, and for medical examinations for employment purposes. Not only are such screening procedures explicitly designed to detect latent ill health and liability to future disease, they also frequently incorporate a genetic dimension. This occurs through requests for information about the past and present diseases of family members. As this procedure has so far, and for the most part, been accepted unquestioningly should there be any unease when more detailed and precise questions about disease predisposition are required? For those disorders inherited through less complex genetic mechanisms, examples exist of conflict between giving individuals easy access to genetic information to assist them in reproductive planning, and the acquisition of this knowledge by insurance companies which refuse mortgage protection and life insurance to the carrier of a malfunctioning gene (Barton 1990). These initial conflicts could escalate, as the ability of genetic testing to predict disease liability for common disorders continues to grow (*Nature* 1990, 1991a, 1991b). Hypertension, for example, clearly has a significant genetic component. The mortality risk from coronary artery disease can be roughly estimated by screening life assurance applicants for raised cholesterol levels. Although none of the insurance companies surveyed by Neil and Mant (1991) required such screening before underwriting life assurance, it seems likely that this situation may change in the near future. There is now good evidence for the involvement of specific genes in some cases of colon and breast cancer (Marx 1990; Ponder 1990). The field of cancer genetics is advancing rapidly, and major strides in disease liability prediction will have been taken by the turn of the century. However most of the future predictions will be of a relatively low probability, perhaps of the order of 10 per cent to 20 per cent, rather than of the virtual certainty of disease which, for example, carriers of the polycystic kidney gene face in relation to renal cysts, even though not all will progress to hypertension or chronic renal failure (Ravine *et al.* 1991).

Screening for genetic conditions raises several major issues especially in relation to its use for insurance purposes. First, the results of genetic screening tests weight the outcome of life insurance unfairly in the insurer's direction. Insurance is fundamentally a gambling proposition, in which the odds will increasingly, and perhaps overwhelmingly in the end, favour the insurers. In such a situation there may be little value in life insurance for many people.

Second, when risks are unclear, insurers spread those risks across those who may have better and those who may have worse health. With the greater ability to predict future health problems – accidents apart – the relevance and the worth of health insurance would simply decrease for affected individuals. Third, insurance contains an 'averaging' element. Knowing which disorders are particularly likely to strike particular individuals does not alter the total aggregate risk borne by insurers, but only its distribution. In principle, improved risk apportionment based on genetic screening should enable insurers to offer better terms to some, whilst loading the premiums of others. How this will work in practice remains to be seen. Already it is expected that insurance companies will protect their clients from others who voluntarily expose themselves to higher risk (e.g. through hazardous hobbies such as smoking or driving a racing car). However genetic predispositions are beyond individual control, and thus raise major additional issues.

Whilst insurers must be protected from unscrupulous clients, many of these issues require early and fundamental public and political debate. They cannot simply be left to insurance companies to formulate relevant policies. It is also not clear that market forces will resolve the situation equitably. It is likely therefore that formal government intervention will prove necessary. Legislation has already been proposed in the Netherlands (EEC Written question no. 566/90, 1990). Legislation has been proposed in Denmark to ban the use of genetic testing for the purposes of employment, pensions and insurance (*Lancet* 1991). A Human Genome Privacy Act has been proposed for the United States (Davies and Gershon 1990), whilst that proposed for California was passed by the State Legislature only to be vetoed by the Governor (Aldhous 1991; Anderson 1991). However none of these solutions seem to address the issue of striking a new balance in the light of current major developments in screening. They are, in the main, attempts to freeze the present situation pending further debate over the rights and duties of the insurer and the insured.

GENE THERAPY

The subject of gene therapy has received substantial media attention, but does not appear to pose major social issues at this time. There is a fundamental distinction between *somatic gene therapy* (attempts to use the genetic manipulation of body cells to correct disorders in an individual, in which the duration of the therapy is limited to the lifespan of that individual, and *germ line therapy*, which attempts to correct a genetic defect in the sperm and egg-producing cells, so that the disease-causing mutation is eliminated from the family line. The question of safety is particularly important in relation to both types of therapy, but it is in principle no different from other questions of safety in medical research and practice.

Somatic gene therapy has already been attempted (with some initial success; see Joyce 1990; Rosenberg *et al.* 1990; Martuza *et al.* 1991) in America, and can be seen as posing no more of a threat than transplant surgery. Germ line therapy is radically different because of its potentially long-lasting effects through many generations. It also raises the worst fears of those who dread a new eugenics movement. However germ line therapy is not yet practicable, and there is agreement that stringent controls are necessary to ensure the safety of the procedures, and of the situations in which they might be used. The prospect of entrepreneurial dictators of the future raising designer bodyguards (or athletes, or classical musicians) is macabre, probably totally impossible, and certainly extremely undesirable.

WHO OWNS GENETIC INFORMATION?

The final issue we wish to address concerns the balance of rights between an individual, and the close members of his or her family, who share many of the same genes. Our genetic endowment is a common heritage. In many situations, at least with current technology, full elucidation of an individual's genetic constitution requires information from family members in order to be able to interpret the genetic data appropriately. For example, in order to evaluate accurately the probability that a young woman is a carrier of muscular dystrophy, it might be necessary to obtain samples from her mother, father, sister and affected nephew. Without this information, she may have to choose between risking that she may produce an affected male child, or terminating all male pregnancies, or remaining childless. It can be argued that the woman has a right to the information (Radcliffe-Richards and Bobrow 1991), but it can only be obtained with the consent of her relatives. A sister or other family member refusing to give a blood sample, from whatever motives, can effectively block the assessment process. This difficult issue raises the question of whether the right to control one's own body includes the right to inflict this form of harm on others – that is whether the 'ownership of genes' is vested entirely in each individual, or has some communality – and is essentially an ethical one (Zimmerli 1990; Radcliffe-Richards and Bobrow 1991). However if the present balance between individual and collective 'ownership' is altered it is likely to require legislation to support the change, and such a change will raise some very significant social issues of freedom and responsibility.

A further issue arising from considering the collective context of screening is the question of privacy. How can we protect an individual's right to keep private the knowledge that he or she will (or will not) develop Huntington's chorea, whilst making use of that knowledge to offer predictive testing to close relatives? How can we ensure that one person's right of access to the information needed to make plans for their life can be achieved without forcing another person to submit to a test they would not wish to take voluntarily? Moreover it is increasingly possible that further research will reveal information about individual genetic susceptibilities in relation to which those individuals may be completely uninformed. In this respect geneticists may become aware that particular people are at risk for a particular disorder, as has been the case with French geneticists studying the family pedigree for some 30,000 living men and women descended from a fifteenth century Breton couple with a history of hereditary juvenile glaucoma (Dorozynski 1991). Should they then invade an individual's privacy by contacting them, uninvited, with this information? May they indeed have a duty to do so (Pelias 1991), regardless of an individual's wishes? These issues, too, need urgent debate.

CONCLUSION

The new biology has considerable power. The mechanics of life – that is how organisms carry out and control their development and daily functions – are being quickly revealed. A great deal will be learnt of direct relevance to ill health and disability. Knowledge is power, and this new knowledge will give the power to develop new therapeutic and preventive strategies. The ability to create proteins tailored to our requirements, and to produce the products of living tissues (such as blood Factor VIII) in the laboratory has already begun to offer remedial therapies. But inevitably such new power brings new responsibility. It is also inevitable (and an important and necessary part of social evaluation) that some who cannot share in the excitement of acquiring, developing or directly using this new knowledge will give more prominence to the problems it brings than to its potential for good. It is equally obvious that some of the scientists involved will, by temperament, not be unduly contemplative of, or sensitive to, genuine public concerns. Many of these concerns are in practice rooted in ignorance of the limitations of the techniques, and in the fear of a much greater power than will really be acquired in this process. However some of the problems raised in public debate are substantial ones, and require real solutions. These solutions must represent a consensus position not unduly dominated either by active proselytizing scientists, or by those who fear that each increment of knowledge is a step into danger. To arrive at a beneficial resolution of these conflicting views requires serious and important social debate.

REFERENCES

Aldhous, P. (1991), 'California tackles insurance', *Nature*, CCCLIII, p. 5
Anderson, C. (1991), 'Privacy bill vetoed', *Nature*, CCCLIII, p. 687
Angastiniotis, M. (1990), 'Cyprus: thalassaemia programme', *Lancet*, CCCXXXVI, pp. 1119–20
Barton, C. J. (1990), 'Hereditary (primary) haemochromatosis', *British Medical Journal*, CCCI, p. 557
Beaudet, A. L. (1990), 'Invited editorial: carrier screening for cystic fibrosis', *American Journal of Medical Genetics*, XLVII, pp. 603–5
Brock, D. J. H., Curtis, A., Mennie, M. and Raeburn, J. A., (1990), 'Options for prenatal testing for Huntington's disease using linked DNA probes', *Journal of Medical Genetics*, XXVII, pp. 68–9
Caskey, C. T., Kaback, M. M., Beaudet, A. L., and Cavalli-Sforza, L. L., (1990), 'The American Society of Human Genetics Statement on Cystic Fibrosis Screening', *American Journal of Human Genetics*, XLVI, p. 393

Davies, K. and Gershon, D. (1990), 'Law to keep labels off genes', *Nature*, CCCXLVII, p. 221

Dorozynski, A. (1991), 'Privacy rules blindside French glaucoma effort', *Science*, CCLII, pp. 369–70

EEC Written question no. 566/90, *Official Journal of the European Communities*, no. c.207/42, 20 August 1990

Frets, P. G., Duivenboorden, H. J., Verhage, F., Peters-Romeyn, B. M. T. and Niermeijer, M. F. (1991), 'Analysis of problems in making the reproductive decision after genetic counselling', *Journal of Medical Genetics*, XXVIII, pp. 194–200

Hodgkinson, K. A., Kerzin-Storrar, L., Watters, E. A. and Harris, R. (1990), 'Adult polycystic kidney disease: knowledge, experience, and attitudes to prenatal diagnosis', *Journal of Medical Genetics*, XXVII, pp. 552–8

Huggins, M., Block N., Kanani, S., Quarrell, O. W. J., Theilman, J., Hedrick, A., Dickens, B., Lynch, A. and Hayden, M. (1990), 'Ethical and legal dilemmas arising during predictive testing for adult-onset disease: the experience of Huntington's disease', *American Journal of Human Genetics*, XLVII, pp. 4–12

Jayaraman, K. S. (1991), 'Saving female babies', *Nature*, CCCLIII, p.594

Journal of Medical Genetics (1990), 'Ethical issues policy statement on Huntington's disease molecular genetics predictive test', XXVII, pp. 34–8

Joyce, C. (1990), 'Four-year-old is first gene therapy patient', *New Scientist*, 22 September 1990, p. 25

Kaback, M. M. (1981), 'Heterozygote screening and prenatal diagnosis in Tay-Sachs disease: a worldwide update', in J. W. Callahan and J. A. Lowden (eds.), *Lysosomes and Lysosomal Storage Disease*, Raven Press, New York pp. 331–42

Kaplan, F., Clow, C. and Scriver, C. R. (1991), 'Cystic fibrosis carrier screening by DNA analysis: a pilot study of attitudes among participants', *American Journal of Human Genetics*, XLIX, pp. 240–41

Lancet (1990), 'Cystic fibrosis: prospects for screening and therapy', CCCXXXV, pp. 79–80

—— (1991), 'Proposed ban on genetic testing in Denmark', CCCXXXVII, p. 1340

Marteau, T. M. (1989), 'Psychological costs of screening', *British Medical Journal*, CCLCLIX, p. 527

—— (1990), 'The need for caution on genetic screening', *New Scientist*, 1747, p. 6

Martuza, R. L., Malick, A., Markert, J. M., Ruffner, K. L. and Coen, D. M. (1991), 'Experimental therapy of human glioma by means of a genetically engineered virus mutant', *Science*, CCLII, pp. 854–6

Marx, J. (1990), 'Genetic defect identified in rare cancer syndrome', *Science*, CCLI, p. 209

Modell, B., Petrou, M., Ward, R. H. T., Fairweather, D. V. I., Rodeck, C., Varnavides, L. A. and White, J. M. (1984), 'Effect of fetal diagnostic testing on the birth-rate of thalassaemia major in Britain', *Lancet*, II, pp. 1383–86

Monk, M. (1991), 'Diagnosis of genetic disease in preimplantation embryos', in J. Lindsten and U. Pettersson (eds.), *Etiology of human disease at the DNA level*, Nobel Symposium 80, Raven Press, New York, pp. 245–60

Nature, (1990), 'Editorial: bad luck insurance', CCCXLVII, p. 214

—— (1991a), 'Editorial: ethics and the human genome', CCCLI, p. 591

—— (1991b), 'Editorial: ethical problems to merit the name', CCCLII, pp. 359–60

Neil, H. A. W. and Mant, D. (1991), 'Cholesterol screening and life assurance', *British Medical Journal*, cccii, pp. 891–3

Ng, I. S. L., Pace, R., Richard, M. V., Kobayashi, Keiko, Kerem, B. S., Tsui, L. C. and Beaudet, A. L. (1991), 'Methods for analysis of multiple cystic fibrosis mutations', *Human Genetics*, lxxxvii, pp. 613–17

Pelias, M. Z. (1991), 'Duty to disclose in medical genetics: a legal perspective', *American Journal of Medical Genetics*, xxxix, pp. 347–54

Ponder, B. A. J. (1990), 'Inherited predisposition to cancer', *Trends in Genetics*, vi-vii, pp. 213–18

Radcliffe-Richards, J. and Bobrow, M. (1991), 'Ethical issues in clinical genetics', *Journal of the Royal College of Physicians*, xxv

Ravine, D., Walker, R. G., Gibson, R. N., Sheffield, L. J., Kincaid-Smith, P. and Danks, D. M. (1991), 'Treatable complications in undiagnosed cases of autosomal dominant polycystic kidney disease', *Lancet*, cccxxxvii, pp. 127–9

Riordan, J. R., Rommens, J. A., Kerem, B., Alon, N., Rozmahel, R., Grzelczak, Z., Zielenski, J., Si, L., Plavsic, N., Chou, J. L., Drumm, M. L., Iannuzzi, M. C., Collins, F. S. and Tsui, L. C. (1989), 'Identification of the cystic fibrosis gene: cloning and characterization of complementary DNA', *Science*, ccxlv, pp. 1066–73

Rosenberg, S. A., Aebersold, P., Cornetta, K., Kasid, A., Morgan, R. A., Moen, R., Karson, E. M., Lotze, M. T., Yang, J. C., Topalian, S. L., Merino, M. J., Culver, K., Miller, A. D., Blaese, R. N. and Anderson, W. F. (1990), 'Gene transfer into humans: immunotherapy of patients with advanced melanoma, using tumor-infiltrating lymphocytes modified by retroviral gene transduction', *New England Journal of Medicine*, cccxxiii, pp. 570–8

Royal College of Physicians (1989), *Prenatal Diagnosis and Genetic Screening: Community and Service Implications*, Royal College of Physicians, London

Rutkow, I. M. and Lipton, J. M. (1974), 'Some negative aspects of state health departments: policies related to screening for sickle cell anemia', *American Journal of Public Health*, lxiv, pp. 217–21

Skraastad, M. O., Verwest, A., Bakker, E., Vegter van der Vlis, M., van Leeuwen-Cornelisse, I., Roos, R. A. C., Pearson, P. L. and van Ommen, G. J. B. (1991), 'Presymptomatic, prenatal, and exclusion testing for Huntington's disease using seven closely linked DNA markers', *American Journal of Medical Genetics*, xxxix, pp. 217–22

Ten Kate, L. P. and Tjimstra, T. (1989), 'Carrier screening for cystic fibrosis', *Lancet* II, 973–4

Weatherall, D. J. (1991), *The New Genetics and Clinical Practice*, 3rd edition, Oxford University Press

Williamson, R., Allison, M. E. D., Bentley, T. J., Lim, S. M. C., Watson, E., Chapple, J., Adam, S. and Boulton, M. (1991), 'Community attitudes to cystic fibrosis carrier testing in England: a pilot study', *Prenatal Diagnosis*, ix, pp. 727–34

World Health Organization (1983), *Progress in Community Control of Thalassaemias*, (Report of the second annual meeting, WHO Working Group on the Community Control of Hereditary Anaemias, World Health Organization, Geneva

Zeesman, S., Clow, C. L., Cartier, L. and Scriver, C. R. (1984), 'A private view of heterozygosity: an eight-year follow-up study on carriers of the Tay-Sachs gene detected by high school screening in Montreal', *American Journal of Medical Genetics*, xviii, pp. 769–78

Zimmerli, W. C. (1990), 'Who has the right to know the genetic constitution of a particular person?', in Chadwick, D., Bock, G. and Whelan, J. (eds.), *Human Genetic Information: Science, Law and Ethics*, CIBA Foundation Symposium 149, Wiley, Chichester, 149, pp. 93–102

3

Screening for foetal and genetic disease: some social and psychological consequences

MARTIN RICHARDS AND JO GREEN

INTRODUCTION

The rapid clinical application of new techniques from biochemistry and molecular genetics has made screening for foetal abnormality and genetic disease the predominant theme of antenatal care in many industrialised countries. The importance of this process lies not only in the particular consequences for individual women and their pregnancies, but also in the more general ways it is changing our perception of pregnancy. This process is changing the relationship between parents and clinicians. As the range of prenatal tests and screening procedures increases, theoretically the choices available to women widen.

However, as we shall see, the evidence suggests that many women are not fully informed about the nature and implications of the tests they undergo in pregnancy. In effect, they do not exercise the choice that is, in theory, available to them. While obstetricians and others involved in deploying tests often argue that they provide reassurance for women, psychological research suggests that they may also cause anxiety (Farrant, 1985; Green, 1990).

The timing of the interventions required to test for the presence of abnormalities, and the associated need for an array of equipment and personnel to implement and assess these techniques has come to shape the pattern of care offered to pregnant women. For a small group of women who enter pregnancy knowing that they have a raised risk of bearing a child with a particular condition these tests offer new possibilities. Such women may have been identified because they have previously had an affected child, or have a family history of a genetic condition. In principle in some of these cases an affected foetus can be identified and aborted so that the pregnant woman and her family can be relieved of the possibility of giving birth to further affected children. In these situations the existence of the new techniques may provide a wider range of options which, for example, lead some couples to embark on further pregnancies which they might have previously avoided. The precise diagnoses which these techniques make possible provide potentially more acceptable reproductive strategies in other situations. In some sex linked conditions, such as Duchenne muscular dystrophy, the birth of an affected child could, until recently, only be avoided by aborting all male foetuses. Now, for many women, prenatal tests allow for the diagnosis of affected foetuses only. Thus terminations can be limited to this group (see Chapter 2). However, the situation for parents who know themselves to be at risk of having a child with a condition that can be diagnosed prenatally is very different from that of the great bulk of the population who have a very small risk of having an abnormal baby. The great majority of this latter group will go through the tests, perhaps expressing anxiety, but learning that the conditions tested for have not been detected. For a very small group there will be the bolt from the blue of being told that an abnormality is present and having to decide whether or not to proceed with the pregnancy.

As well as the consequences for particular couples who have a high risk of having a child with a particular disorder, or those who unexpectedly are told that something is wrong, more general social effects of the new screening techniques have been claimed. It has been suggested that the recent increase in the fertility of women aged 35 years and older is, in part, the result of the availability of prenatal screening and diagnostic techniques which can be used to avoid the increased risk of the birth of children with certain abnormalities, such as Down's syndrome, which occurs with rising maternal age. However, others argue that such changes must be set in the context of broader demographic changes which have, in particular, changed attitudes towards, as well as the economic and social possibilities, of later pregnancies and that the direct effects of prenatal screening and diagnosis are likely to be very small.

The consequences of new screening and diagnostic procedures must, however, be considered in relation to a series of uncertainties and problems which currently attend their use. Most obviously, virtually all the conditions that can be identified in pregnancy are currently untreatable. All that can be offered to prospective parents is the possibility of screening, diagnosis and abortion. Given that most pregnancies are normal, most parents will suffer the inconvenience and anxieties associated with the procedure for no gain, save that of knowing that some disorders are not present. Prenatal screening and diagnosis are relatively expensive. In countries such as Britain where the overall health budget is more or less limited, development of these services is likely to lead to the reduction of other provision of care. Neither screening nor diagnostic tests offer complete accuracy. Whilst errors in the detection of the targeted abnormality may be rare, the effects of such errors can be devastating for the families involved. Parents often are not fully informed about inaccuracies and so may find a false positive or false negative result more distressing than it might have been had they better understood what the procedure entailed.

But above all screening and diagnosis is only possible for a limited number of serious foetal conditions so the techniques detect a small group of abnormalities, rather than ensuring, as some may be led to believe, the birth of a healthy baby. Indeed, at a population level, the impact that screening techniques have had so far on the prevalence of serious disability resulting from congenital abnormalities has been minimal. Overall, approximately 3–4 per cent of pregnancies are affected by a congenital abnormality but many of these cannot be identified by current techniques. Thus whilst the speed with which the structure of the human genome is being unravelled is increasing considerably, and the specific genetic loci of some of the more common and intractable genetic diseases are being revealed with gathering pace, the range of abnormalities detectable through prenatal diagnosis still remains small. And, of course, many abnormalities are not associated with specific gene defects. For the vast majority of pregnant women who are not known to be at particular risk, the chance of identifying an affected foetus through prenatal screening is small (Wald, 1984; Chard and Macintosh, 1992). It is on these women that we focus in this chapter.

THE NATURE AND AVAILABILITY OF PRENATAL SCREENING AND DIAGNOSTIC TECHNOLOGIES

Amniocentesis has for some years been the major prenatal diagnostic procedure used to detect a range of genetic abnormalities. Traditionally carried out in the fourth month of pregnancy it can be used to detect Down's syndrome and other abnormalities, as well as the sex of the foetus, from cultured foetal cells from the amniotic fluid. It can also provide amniotic fluid which can be analysed biochemically to detect other abnormalities. However the complexity, cost and general resource implications of the procedure have led to considerable pressure to develop less intrusive, earlier tests, a process accelerated by concern about miscarriages occurring in approximately 0.5 per cent of cases through the use of this procedure.

Since the 1980s chorionic villus sampling has been developed, and increasingly deployed, in the hope that the procedure would offer similar results to amniocentesis but substantially earlier in a pregnancy. Chorionic villus sampling (CVS) involves sampling cells from the membrane which surrounds the foetus, and is usually undertaken before the twelfth week of pregnancy. The value of earlier diagnosis, and if necessary an earlier and, perhaps, less traumatic, abortion is important (Chard and Macintosh, 1992), however the clinical accuracy of CVS is currently lower than that of amniocentesis, and the procedure is associated with higher rates of miscarriage and possibly with foetal deformities in some situations.

Given the risks, complications and costs of these techniques, they are usually only offered to women known to be at an increased risk of the relevant conditions. Apart from those with a previous history, this group may be defined by maternal age (usually over 35) or by the results of a biochemical serum (blood) screening test. For some foetal abnormalities the levels of biochemical 'markers' can be used to assign a probability that a foetus is affected. So for Down's syndrome previous policies can thus be refined so that now, in principle, all women can be biochemically tested, and amniocenteses can now be restricted to those identified through biochemical tests as having a significant risk of a foetus with Down's syndrome. Although it is the case that the risk of a Down's child for an individual woman is higher with increasing age, the majority of Down's births have been occurring to younger women (under age 35) because of the greater absolute numbers of births amongst this group who are not usually offered amniocentesis or CVS. Now, in principle at least, all women can be given a serum screening test – which is relatively simple and cheap – and only those at an increased risk be offered amniocentesis. Such a policy should in principle lead to the diagnosis of a significant number of foetuses with Down's syndrome in younger women and reduce the need for amniocentesis for those in the older group (at least for this indication). However as yet it is unclear whether or not such benefits are being realised.

As ultrasound techniques have been further developed to allow an apparently more accurate visualisation of the foetus, their use for screening and diagnosis of abnormality has now become routine, extending far beyond their earlier use for dating pregnancies and charting foetal growth rates. 'Structural anomaly scans' are carried out at around 19 weeks of gestation in many maternity hospitals in Britain. False positive and false negative results are not uncommon. In addition, there is evidence that there is a discrepancy between the way that women and their families perceive and use the results of the scans, and the ways in which they are clinically perceived (Green *et al.*, 1993c). Whilst women generally see the scans as confirmation that they have a healthy baby, clinically they are viewed as a way of seeking out abnormality. Such discrepancies in the way that scans have been perceived may lead to serious misunderstanding between parents and clinicians. The operation of the scans in 'real time' may also produce further difficulties. Parents like them because they can 'see' the baby and watch its movements. However, should an apparent abnormality be found which often will result in the need to bring in other clinicians to confirm a suspicion, considerable skills of stage management and communication are required to convey the news to the mother without arousing unnecessary anxieties. It is unusual within medicine for a diagnosis to have to be made quite so literally in front of the patient, or at least its mother.

THE SOCIAL AND PSYCHOLOGICAL EFFECTS OF SCREENING AND PRENATAL DIAGNOSIS

There is now a considerable body of research on the social and psychological aspects of prenatal screening and diagnosis (e.g. Green, 1990; 1994; Green *et al.*, 1992; 1993a, b, c; Farrant, 1985; Lippman, *et al.*, 1985; Marteau *et al.*, 1989; Richards, 1989; Richards and Green, 1993). This work has explored many aspects of the impact of the new technologies including their uptake; pregnant women's knowledge of them; the extent to which their use may be reassuring or anxiety provoking; the communication of test results, and the analysis of attitudes towards abortion. Other research has been more descriptive aiming to capture women's experience undergoing or contemplating prenatal diagnosis or screening (Green *et al.*, 1992; Marteau, *et al.*, 1993; Rothman, 1986). In this chapter we will concentrate on four topics which are of special importance when considering the impact of the new technologies. These are: the knowledge of risk associated both with procedures and the conditions to which they relate; women's understanding and attitudes towards the termination of pregnancy; the attitudes of providers and recipients of the screening and diagnostic services; and issues of information and consent associated with these technologies.

THE SOCIAL CONTEXT OF PRENATAL DIAGNOSIS AND WOMEN'S KNOWLEDGE OF RISK

As we have already pointed out, prenatal testing for foetal abnormality has a very different meaning for the relatively small number of women who know themselves to be at risk before the investigative procedures begin compared to the great majority of women who may perceive their risk status to be low. The former group is likely to be well informed about the condition for which their foetus has increased risk; is likely to know about the relevant test procedures; and will probably have already experienced them, and their costs and benefits. Usually parents in such a difficult situation – possibly already with a living child with the condition – will have considered whether to take the appropriate tests before the pregnancy, and may have decided, if the tests are positive, whether to have an abortion. For such parents the question of whether the new pregnancy will be of a normal child, or another with the same condition is likely to affect their approach to all the antenatal procedures.

For the great majority of parents who have no reason to believe that they are at risk the situation is very different. For most such women and their partners there is little appreciation of the potential consequences of foetal screening, for it is perceived as simply a part of the series of routines that constitute antenatal care, and may well also be considered by those undergoing such care as a means of further confirming the healthy status of their baby. Indeed, the pattern of tests is often presented to pregnant women in a way that encourages a routine and benign view of the status of these interventions in pregnancy (Richards and Green, 1993; Marteau *et al.*, 1992).

The context within which most women undertake prenatal screening and diagnostic tests is extremely important in interpreting the relatively routine way in which they are treated. Antenatal care is unusual, indeed in many ways quite extraordinary, amongst procedures of a preventive nature in medicine in that it has an extremely high uptake. Virtually all pregnant women in Britain use antenatal clinics and attendance is largely taken for granted as a necessary preliminary to the birth (Richards and Green, 1993). Indeed, a recent study has shown that most women believe that regular attendance at antenatal clinics is *essential* (Green *et al.*, 1993c). The system of care which is offered to women is taken up almost universally and is virtually unquestioned. One reason for this situation is very obvious: women have been persuaded that it is in their interest, and above all in the interest of their babies, to follow unequivocally the medical procedures which are presented to them as desirable by doctors, midwives, and others professionally concerned with the management of pregnancy and childbirth.

The history of antenatal care and the way it has developed as an integral part of maternity care has contributed to its taken-for- granted character for most mothers. As Oakley (1982) and others have described, obstetricians have managed to enshrine a medical definition of pregnancy so that its fusion with medical procedures has become routine. The progress of the pregnancy for women as well as for clinical staff is marked by the schedule of antenatal visits and events such as the ultrasound scan at which a woman first 'sees' her baby.

Research on women's perception of prenatal screening and diagnosis confirms that the new techniques are usually perceived as an integral part of more traditional antenatal care and are accepted within this framework. The research of Marteau *et al.* (1989) shows, for example, that many women just accept the pattern of care which they have been offered, and may not recall the particular tests to which they have been subject, nor have any idea about their potential significance. Such perceptions are encouraged by the way in which the tests are offered. For example, in one study a midwife said to a mother that 'if you want a happy, healthy baby then you'll have the test' (Green *et al.*, 1992). As MacIntyre (1987) first noted, the widely used but ambiguous phrase, a test 'to make sure your baby is alright', allows women to view almost any procedure as one that may help to ensure normality rather than to detect abnormality.

Further support for the view that prenatal screening has become part of the taken-for-granted package of antenatal care is that it now seems of little consequence to many mothers whether or not they are given the results of any particular tests, as Green *et al.* (1993c) found with maternal serum alpha-fetoprotein screening (AFP). While this taken-for-granted attitude means that women are not made anxious by test procedures, it also means that they may fail to derive any reassurance from their results (Green *et al.* 1993c). Since for most women, reassurance is the most likely benefit of undertaking the procedures, and indeed may be the primary motivation for undergoing testing (Farrant, 1985), this is an important loss. Furthermore, the fact that many women undergo screening procedures with little understanding of what they are, or what their implications might be, raises important questions about the nature of their initial consent. This issue is pursued further below.

The termination of pregnancy and prenatal tests
The only 'treatment' that can currently be offered for most genetic abnormalities and their associated and subsequent diseases, apart from care and some symptomatic management, is an abortion. This possibility is offered to, and accepted by, women in the great majority of cases in which positive test results are given (see Green *et al.*, 1993a). Only a very small number of parents decide to proceed with a pregnancy once a diagnosis is made, even when the abnormality is relatively mild as, for example, in certain sex chromosome abnormalities.

Under the Human Fertilization and Embryology Act 1991, the law in England and Wales was changed to allow abortions on the grounds of risk to the mother's life or health, or when 'there is a substantial risk that if the child were born it would suffer from such physical or mental abnormality as to be seriously disabled' at any point in pregnancy up to term. As legal commentators have noted (e.g. Morgan, 1992) neither parliament nor the courts have shown much interest in trying to define more precisely what is meant by 'serious disability' resulting in great confusion for parents and clinicians.

Abortions for reasons of foetal abnormality are rare and only make up about 2 per cent of the total carried out in England and Wales. Whilst some professionals may still believe that such abortions are easier for parents to cope with because they are for a 'good reason', the evidence suggests that this is not the case. Indeed they are particularly distressing to women and may have long term consequences. The crisis they engender is comparable to that suffered after a perinatal death (e.g. Lloyd and Lawrence, 1985; Statham, 1992) for which adequate counselling and support is often not available.

An important issue that must be raised here is social attitudes towards disabled people and those who care for them. It is a hard and continuing struggle to ensure that adequate services and support are available to disabled people in a climate where government policies are re-evaluating all forms of social welfare benefits. Whilst public attitudes towards disabled people may have become more accepting and positive in recent decades, not least through lobbying and action by such people themselves, how are such attitudes going to be affected by the ready access to abortion for abnormalities disclosed in pregnancy? It is also important to note that, as with other medical and health services, the take-up of prenatal screening and diagnosis is not equitably distributed across the social spectrum. Some socially and economically disadvantaged women do not enter the antenatal care system until late in pregnancy, and so may not have prenatal screening or diagnosis. The effect of such factors may be that an increasing proportion of abnormal foetuses will be carried by mothers in disadvantaged groups, which also include many ethnic minorities (see Knott *et al.*, 1986). In this situation it may be that those least able to provide for children with disabilities will be those most likely to bear them.

The attitudes of providers and recipients of prenatal screening and diagnosis
As has been discussed earlier, there are significant differences between the attitudes and approaches of the providers and recipients of pre-natal screening services. For most women the primary goal of prenatal screening is reassurance that all is well with their babies, whilst obste-tricians place priority on the detection of abnormalities, and the abortion of affected foetuses. These attitudes have led to some obste-tricians restricting screening and diagnosis to women who will make a prior commitment to abort in the event of a positive diagnosis. This difference between the perspective of the provider and the user of the service is also illustrated by Farrant's (1985) finding that, whilst 80 per cent of obstetricians rated the communication of a positive diagnosis as very urgent, only 23 per cent gave the same priority to a negative result. This attitude also leads some obstetricians not to inform women at all about negative results and simply to tell them they may assume that all is well if they do not hear anything by a particular date – a strategy that has been shown to be especially effective in creating anxiety (Fearn *et al.*, 1982). These same attitudes may be responsible for the low priority given to the provision of counselling services compared to the screening and diagnostic proce-dures themselves and abortion facilities.

In public, service providers usually claim that prenatal screening offers choice to women and their families. But this position is belied by the way in which services are offered. Certain choices are not deemed ethically appropriate. For example, couples are not permitted in Britain to use prenatal diagnostic techniques to ensure the birth of a baby of a preferred sex. Within the health services, rather than in public debate, screening programmes are usually justified by cost-benefit analyses which indicate the costs that will be saved in terms of the long term care and support that would have been needed for a disabled child. This, too, is the approach which usually governs how the performance of screening programmes is assessed – by the numbers of affected foetuses detected and their fate. We are unaware of any clinical attempt to evaluate a prenatal screening programme by assessing the benefits that *parents* might gain, or the extent to which increased choice might be welcomed by recipients of the tests.

Clearly prenatal screening, like clinical genetics, operates in the shadow of the history of eugenics. The attempts to encourage the reproduction of the fittest members of society and to discourage reproduction among the least fit which was such a prominent part of social policy in the early part of the century and a preoccupation amongst many interested in human genetics (Kevles, 1985) became increasingly disreputable by the late 1930s. Discomfort about history has stifled the debate that ought to have taken place about the ways in which prenatal screening and diagnosis should or should not be developed. Symptomatic of this was the reaction to a recent article by a geneticist who claimed in the *Lancet* that 'ostensibly non-directive counselling in connection with prenatal diagnosis is inevitably a sham, not because of a personal failure on the part of the genetic counsellor, but as a direct result of the structure of the encounter between counsellor and client' (Clarke, 1991). This statement drew a sharp retort from a senior clinical geneticist that the 'reduction of the birth incidence of genetic disorders is not the object of genetic services' (Pembrey, 1991).

However, prenatal screening is often accepted by parents as part of an antenatal care package. Many of those who are screened have little idea of what is happening to them and its implications. They seek reassurance and are pleased to have a test that will 'make sure your baby is alright'. For the few who receive a positive test result and the news that their baby has an abnormality, it may be very difficult to refuse the offer of an abortion. Therefore, choice is, in effect, very limited for those who are recipients of the screening tests. A positive diagnosis for a congenital abnormality will, by and large, lead to the abortion of a foetus. Yet, there has been very little public debate about the conditions for which it is and is not appropriate to screen. In relation to some conditions, such as males with an extra Y chromosome, it seems very unlikely that a specific screening programme would be set up as those with the condition usually lead completely normal lives and most are quite unaware of their chromosomal status. However, this condition will be revealed when chromosomes are examined for other purposes (such as the diagnosis of Down's syndrome), and it appears that this information is usually passed to parents. The result is usually the abortion of an XYY foetus, despite the more or less normal outcome for those with this condition.

Creating an appropriate context for giving information about prenatal diagnosis and screening

There is a major dilemma in relation to prenatal diagnosis and screening. As we have described, while the majority of women do not see themselves at any particular risk, they accept prenatal screening without question, or without great concern, as part of the antenatal care package (Green *et al.*, 1992; Marteau *et al.*, 1989). For the very small minority for whom the news is bad, there is no chance to prepare themselves for this eventuality and, typically, they proceed to an abortion as the only choice available to them. But for the majority, their lack of knowledge about the testing process and what it might lead to protects them from worry and anxiety. But it can be argued that the majority of women *do not* give informed consent to the testing to which they are subjected. Should we therefore provide more information about testing and its potential consequences to all pregnant women? To go down this route would almost certainly lead to much more anxiety about such tests in a population where there is a statistically very small chance of an abnormality being detected. In the present situation, in effect, information is restricted and therefore anxiety minimised. Such a policy has obvious personal and social costs. Those who are found to have abnormal foetuses receive such information without warning and, as a consequence, their potential choices in this situation may be reduced. There has also been little public debate about the conditions for which screening should or should not be undertaken. In general, existing screening programmes have been driven by those who develop the tests whose emphasis has been on what is technically and logistically possible, rather than on the personal and social consequences of such programmes. Ways need to be found of opening wider public debate about the nature and context of screening programmes. This may only be done by providing more information about screening and its potential consequences to *all* pregnant women. Such an approach is likely, at least in the short term, to create a higher level of anxiety with a correspondingly greater need to ensure that appropriate counselling and support are available. Inevitably such a strategy would have both additional financial, and further psychological costs. Nonetheless unless that strategy is pursued important decisions are being removed from individual parents about whether they have children, and what kind of children they may have, as well as pre-empting decisions about the broader social consequences of screening and prenatal testing programmes.

ACKNOWLEDGEMENT

The Cambridge Prenatal Screening Project has been funded by the Health Promotion Research Trust to whom our thanks are due.

REFERENCES

Chard, T. and Macintosh, M. (1992), 'Antenatal diagnosis of congenital abnormalities', in T. Chard and M. P. M. Richards, (eds.), *Obstetrics in the 1990s: Current Controversies*, Clinics in Developmental Medicine 123/124. Mackeith Press, London

Clarke, A. (1991), 'Is non-directive genetic counselling possible?', *The Lancet*, 338, pp. 998–1001

Farrant, W. (1985), ' "Who's for amniocentesis?". The politics of prenatal screening', in H. Homans (ed.), *The Sexual Politics of Reproduction*, Gower, London

Fearn, J., Hibbard, B. M., Lawrence, K. M., Roberts, H. and Robinson, J. O. (1982), 'Screening for neural-tube defects and maternal anxiety', *British Journal of Obstetrics and Gynaecology*. 89, pp. 218–21

Green, J. M. (1990), *Calming or Harming? A Critical Review of Psychological Effects of Foetal Diagnosis on Pregnant Women*, Galton Institute Occasional Papers, Second Series No. 2, London

Green, J. M. (1994), 'Women's experiences of prenatal screening and diagnosis', in L. Abramsky, and J. Chapple, J. (eds.), *Prenatal Diagnosis: the Human Side*, Chapman and Hall, London

Green, J. M., Statham, H. and Snowdon, C. (1992), 'Screening for fetal abnormalities: attitudes and experiences', in T. Chard, and M. P. M. Richards, (eds.), *Obstetrics in the 1990s: Current Controversies*, Clinics in Developmental Medicine 123/124. Mackeith Press, London

—— (1993a), 'Pregnant women's attitudes to abortion and prenatal screening', *Journal of Reproductive and Infant Psychology*, 11, pp. 31–40

—— (1993b), Women's knowledge of prenatal screening tests 1: Relationship with hospital screening policy and demographic factors', *Journal of Reproductive and Infant Psychology*, 11, pp. 11–20

—— (1993c), *Pregnancy: A Testing Time*, Report of the Cambridge Prenatal Screening Study, Centre for Family Research, University of Cambridge

Hyde, B. (1986), 'An interview study of pregnant women's attitudes to ultrasound scanning', *Social Science and Medicine*, 22, pp. 587–2

Kevles, D. J. (1985), *In the Name of Eugenics: Genetics and the Uses of Human Heredity*, Knopf, New York

Knott, P. D., Penketh, R. J. A. and Lucas, M. K. (1986), 'Uptake of amniocentesis in women aged 38 years or more: a retrospective study', *British Journal Obstetrics and Gynaecology*, 3, pp. 1246–50

Lippman, A., Perry, T. B., Mandel, S. and Cartier, S. (1985), 'Chorionic villi sampling: women's attitudes', *American Journal of Medical Genetics*, 22, pp. 395–401

Lloyd, J. and Laurence, K. M. (1985), 'Sequelae and support after termination of pregnancy for fetal malformation,' *British Medical Journal*, 290, pp. 907–9

MacIntyre, S. (1987), *Women's Experiences and Attitudes to Screening*, Paper given at King's Fund Forum on Screening for Foetal and Genetic Abnormality, Regent's College, London

Marteau, T. M., Johnston, M., Shaw, R. W. and Slack, J. (1989), 'Factors influencing the uptake of screening for open neural tube defects and amniocentesis to test for Down's syndrome', *British Journal of Obstetrics and Gynaecology*, 96, pp. 739–41

Marteau, T. M., Slack, J., Kidd, J. and Shaw. R. W. (1992), 'Presenting a routine screening test in antenatal care: practice observed', *Public Health*, 106, pp. 131–41

Marteau, T. M., Plenicar, M. and Kidd, J. (1993), 'Obstetricians presenting amniocentesis to pregnant women: practice observed', *Journal of Reproductive and Infant Psychology*, 11, pp. 3–10

Morgan, D. (1992) 'Judges on delivery: change, continuity and regulation in obstetric practice', in T. Chard and M. P. M. Richards, (eds.), *Obstetrics in the 1990s: Current Controversies*, Clinics in Developmental Medicine 123/124, Mackeith Press, London

Oakley, A. (1982), 'The origin and development of antenatal care', in M. Enkin and I. Chalmers, (eds.), *Effectiveness and Satisfaction in Antenatal Care*, Clinics in Developmental Medicine, No. 81/82, SIMP, London

Pembrey, M. (1991), 'Non-directive genetic counselling', *The Lancet* (letter), 338, pp. 1266–67

Richards, M. P. M. (1989), 'Social and ethical problems of foetal diagnosis and screening', *Journal of Reproductive and Infant Psychology*, 7, pp. 171–85

Richards, M. P. M. and Green, J. M. (1993), 'Attitudes toward prenatal screening for foetal abnormality and the detection of carriers of genetic disease: a discussion paper', *Journal of Reproductive and Infant Psychology*, 11, pp. 49–56

Rothman, B. K. (1986), *The Tentative Pregnancy*, Viking, New York

Statham, H. (1992) Professional understanding and parents' experiences of termination', In D. J. Brock, C. H. Rodeck and M. A. Ferguson-Smith (eds.), *Prenatal Screening and Diagnosis*, Churchill Livingston, London, pp. 697–702

Tsoi, M. M. and Hunter, M. (1987), 'Ultrasound scanning in pregnancy: consumer reactions', *Journal of Reproductive and Infant Psychology*, 5, pp. 43–4

Wald, N. J. (1984) *Antenatal and Neonatal Screening*, Oxford University Press

4

The Human Genome Project: creator of the potentially sick, potentially vulnerable and potentially stigmatized?

REGINA KENEA

INTRODUCTION

A story going around Moscow in the late 1970s evokes an interesting aspect of the ethical and social debate surrounding the Human Genome Initiative (HGI). Members of a visiting American dance troupe were very upset about a major problem they faced and sought help from the theatre manager. When he asked what the problem was, they pointed to a big hole in the stage floor. The manager shrugged and said 'That is no problem, that is a detail.'

While awareness of the social, ethical and legal implications of the Human Genome Project (HGP) is high, some scientists supporting the project also seem to regard these concerns as being merely technical details of application. Furthermore, they complain that the 'undue' emphasis on them over complicates discussion about the project and thus prejudices the more important business of pursuing the science. Phrases such as 'scientifically illiterate,' 'misconception' and 'correct perspective' used in the following accounts are revealing and unsettling in their emphasis on the legitimacy and primacy of a particular view of the project.

> It would be a tragedy if 'slippery slope' arguments or misconceptions about what the genome project might tell us about how to manipulate human behaviour were to set back progress in a field which may have more to offer human well-being than almost any in the history of medical and biological research.
>
> (Weatherall, August 1991 p. 30)

> This misconception rests on a failure to distinguish between basic research, the *pure search* for knowledge, and technology, which is the application of that knowledge to practical human affairs.
>
> (Nossal 1990 p. 2, italics added)

> The development of powerful new diagnostic approaches will expand the repertoire of tests available; viewed from the *correct perspective*, this is an advance rather than a source of new problems.
>
> (European Scientific Foundation 1991 p. 19, italics added)

The unfortunate use of 'confused,' and 'misconception,' to portray versions of reality differing from that of the scientists gives the impression that the scientists' version is the objective truth, rather than a particular paradigm that was legitimated in the past and is now being questioned. This language tends to hamper the public airing of social, ethical and legal apprehensions, a necessary step in reaching social consensus in an area of research that can fundamentally alter social norms, institutions and relationships. Societies appear to be cyclical in the domain in which their search for answers lies – from the profane to the spiritual and from the biological to the social. In the United States and most other western countries, biological answers have gained ascendancy.

Clinical geneticists have been extremely successful in portraying medical advances as ways of reducing suffering and conquering disease for specific individuals and families who face the threat of extremely handicapping and possibly lethal diseases. And who can disagree with these goals! Latent negative social effects of such research, however, tend to be ignored. Dialogue about the social dimensions of genetics should be on stage rather than backstage, in relation to which the following questions are pertinent.

1. How will social norms incorporate 'probabilistic' information concerning the rights of the individual in an era depicted by changing concepts of health and disease?
2. How will the advances accruing from the HGP influence how individuals think about themselves and others, relate to one another, and perceive their responsibilities and obligations to significant others as well as to the community at large?
3. How will social norms regarding privacy and control over self- identity evolve, and will the concept of 'inner privacy' be eroded?

These issues may be profitably addressed in terms of the potentially sick, the potentially vulnerable and the potentially stigmatized. However, in order to put the discussion into perspective, debates surrounding the goals and scope of the (HGI) and related social, ethical and legal issues need to be described.

WHAT IS THE HUMAN GENOME PROJECT?

The HGP is a plan to map and sequence all the human genes. So far fewer than 2,000 of the estimated 50,000 to 100,000 genes in the human genome have been mapped onto chromosomes and less than 1 per cent of the entire length of human DNA has been sequenced (National Centre for Human Genome Research) (NCHGR pamphlet, no date). Scientists plan to develop two kinds of chromosome maps – genetic linkage maps and physical maps.

Genetic linkage maps involve studying how frequently individual diseases and other traits are inherited together within families over several generations. Advances in molecular genetics allow scientists to use 'markers' (unique segments of DNA) that can be followed in families as landmarks on a genetic map. If they lie close to the yet unidentified gene suspected of causing the disease, they are likely to be inherited together. Physical maps give the actual distances between genes on a chromosome. It is not enough to know where the genes are located; it is necessary to understand their precise functioning. Determining the order of the nucleotides in the DNA of a gene is known as sequencing, and this order determines the genetic information the gene carries.

The HGP is 'Big Science' in terms of human and monetary resources. The mapping and sequencing of the human genome is likely to generate more data than any other single project in the development of biology as an academic field (European Science Foundation 1991 p. 12). The US government, mainly through the NCHGR at the National Institutes of Health and the Department of Energy (DOE), is expected to fund up to 200 million dollars per year for fifteen years on the project. This work will be carried out internationally. The Human Genome Organization (HUGO), established in 1988, is an international consortium of molecular biologists aimed at ensuring international cooperation, negotiating overlapping interests and sharing knowledge worldwide. Eight countries: the United States, Denmark, France, Germany, Italy, the United Kingdom, Japan, and the former Soviet Union have established national genome projects for which funding has been committed. An additional seven countries – Australia, Canada, Chile, Korea, the Netherlands, New Zealand and Sweden are contemplating, or planning, to initiate national genome programmes. Cooperative research endeavours also are being planned in Latin America and the Nordic countries (European Science Foundation 1991 p. 6).

The objective of the HGI is to improve human existence through spin-off benefits to medicine, biological research, and biotechnology. Yet these 'benefits' may also involve controversial uses of genetic information and technical innovations. Therefore, to anticipate ethical, legal and social issues and to develop policy options addressing them (and placate critics), the NCHGR and DOE will use at least 3 per cent of their annual HGI budgets for scholarly and educational activities pertaining to possible controversial possibilities. Funding for these activities will be provided by the Ethical, Legal and Social Implications (ELSI) programme. HUGO also plans 'to encourage public debate and provide the information and advice on the scientific, ethical, social, legal and commercial implications of human genome projects.' (European Science Foundation, 1991 p. 11)

SOCIAL, ETHICAL AND LEGAL DISCOURSE

Much of the early interdisciplinary debate about the HGP focused on whether doing this project was a good idea, or not, and if it was a good idea, how bad applications could be prevented. Now that the project has been started, interest is focused on the more distant eugenic, evolutionary and 'designer genes' implications; on the more immediate ethical problems posed by future genetic screening tests and by possible clinical use of the new information and techniques, and on protection of the individual from abuses (Andrews and Jaeger 1991; Bobrow and Manners 1994; Gostin, 1991). This emphasis on more immediate problems is reflected in the NCHGR programme on the ELSI of the HGP which identified three priority issues:

1. Privacy of genetic information, including questions of clinical confidentiality and data management.
2. Effective clinical integration of new genetic testing options, including questions of quality control and professional liability.
3. Fairness in the use of genetic information, including questions of insurance availability and employment screening.

Source: (NCHGR 1991 p. 1)

These are essential priorities. But too few investigations have been undertaken into a larger, more subtle, field of inquiry – the effects of applied biomedical technology on the character of society, its social institutions and its culture (Lock 1994; Strathern 1994). Researchers dissect the impact of the HGI on clients and involved professionals but neglect the social and cultural contexts. Yet it is the structural and cultural characteristics of a society which influence the rate at which technological diffusion occurs and the extent to which it is accepted and incorporated.

WHO ARE THE POTENTIALLY SICK, POTENTIALLY VULNERABLE AND POTENTIALLY STIGMATIZED?

The potentially sick, potentially vulnerable and potentially stigmatized are not an esoteric group of people. They are all of us waiting for our harmful genes to be identified. Everyone carries several deleterious genes. By chance, some of us will be identified early and some later; some of us will not have to wait long for a treatment or cure to be found after diagnostic and predictive tests are developed. But the gap may not close for others within their lifetimes (Friedmann 1989; 1990). For most of us, the interaction of genetic and environmental variables will be complex with the accuracy of predictions uncertain (Gostin 1991; Holtzman 1989).

> The elucidation of the genetic component of the common diseases of Western society will undoubtedly take longer and will *require a considerable amount of good luck and ingenuity.* Although it seems likely that steady progress will be made it may be many years before the information gained from these studies has a major impact on clinical practice.
> (Weatherall 1991 p. 28,italics added)

While genetic research is probably inevitable, is the application of newly acquired genetic information inevitable? Is the availability of knowledge implicitly coercive? Zimmerly (1990) disagrees with the assumption that it is impossible to suppress or decline to apply existing knowledge; he claims that the whole history of science and technology is full of examples of such suppression.

> In my opinion, the only reasonable way of thinking about the future in a scientifically and/or philosophically sound manner is to map the possibilities and to make a deliberate choice between them according to their relative feasibility and desirability, of course, by doing so, you inevitably suppress all the others. It is therefore unavoidable that one suppresses possible truths by merely trying to follow one of the possibilities which you regard as true, and which afterwards turns out to be one of the previously mentioned errors or failures.
> (Zimmerly 1990 pp. 78–9)

While history may be full of such suppressions, it is also filled with examples of pressure to use those advances that had not been suppressed but were supported by vested interests. The impetus to develop new information and techniques is to be able to use them or apply them. Furthermore, 'the tendency of the fruits of technological invention [is] to acquire a force of their own and, as it were, make themselves independent of their makers' (Jonas 1985 p. 491).

Much of the increased cost of health care in the United States today is due to the overuse of tests and procedures based both on the fear of malpractice suits and on the sometimes unsubstantiated faith in hi-tech medicine; examples include the regular use of the electronic foetal monitor, and of caesarian sections (Shy +*et al*. 1990; Hurst and Summey 1984). What have been suppressed here are the non- technical options!

Many of the new biotechnologies have made the 'unknowable' knowable. Is this necessarily beneficial? Advances in genetic knowledge discovered by the HGP can lead to a substantial redefinition of the concepts of health, self-identity and privacy in a world consisting of the potentially sick, potentially vulnerable and potentially stigmatized. How can the use of probability as a predictor of future genetic diseases affect our lives and the kind of society in which we live?

Probability as predictor: blurring the distinction between health and disease
Clinical medicine will be increasingly based on probabilities, rather than on certainties. What will the difference be between health and illness, and how will this determination influence physician training and ideas about the human body? Will the concept of a phenotype become outmoded and images of DNA sequences and the double helix be substituted?

Prediction based on probability in clinical medicine, particularly when based on complex genetic inheritance patterns, involves a high risk that both clients and the larger society will internalize misinformation. The first difficulty arises from the erroneous assumption that prediction and probability are the same thing.

> In the genetic field, we should distinguish between the probabilistic expectation, like a 25 per cent chance that you might develop a particular disease some time in the future and the frequency expectation, of 25 per cent of genetic segregation of a homozygote in the case of two heterozygotes. We need to distinguish carefully between probabilistic and predictive medicine.
>
> (Brenner 1990 p. 31)

This is certainly a valid distinction for the scientific community to make, but it is far too difficult to convey accurately to the general public. The public will learn of the uncertainty involved and, perhaps, that the predictions are based on a probability estimate. But people tend to view the world as deterministic, not probabilistic, and schools do not teach children to learn the judgment and decision strategies required for dealing with a probabilistic world. More often, certainty equals security and uncertainty includes an element of fear (Kenen 1994). Another difficulty arises from the uncertainties on which the predictions are based. Today most morbidity and mortality in developed countries is attributed to non-infectious diseases, and most of these are caused by multiple factors. There is no intervention on the horizon that is likely to eliminate non-infectious diseases by aiming at a single aetiological factor in the way that immunizations and antibiotics conquered infectious diseases (Holtzman 1989). To complicate matters further, different combinations of factors affect individuals differently. The expression or penetration of these factors can also vary widely – from full blown manifestations to the absence of clinical symptoms – depending upon whether still unknown factors are absent or present. Yet, despite this known variability, a test report is too often accepted at face value and acted upon, if a probability estimate is attached to it or a 'positive' or 'negative' result is indicated (Nelkin and Tancredi 1989). The willingness to accept a test report as being more precise than it may be, seems to offer an almost mystical sense of reassurance when compared with the alternative of accepting a world of uncertainty.

The difficulty people have in understanding and dealing with probability combined with the uncertainties attached to prognosis pose problems for the medical profession and the larger society. Recombinant DNA technology will lead to the identification of susceptibility-conferring or disease-causing genes for a large number of diseases, and ways to test whether healthy individuals possess these genes will be discovered. Problems with such testing involve the low sensitivity of available tests; counselling dilemmas due to currently unresolvable uncertainty over test results; high costs; confusion and social pressure leading to ill thought out reproductive decisions; and the lack of pilot studies carried out on the benefit of using carrier testing. Such difficulties have led to the recommendation *not* to undertake a population screening programme for cystic fibrosis in the United States at the present time (Beaudet 1990).

Future health providers will test patients for genetic abnormalities and then try to categorize them as being either healthy or sick. Individuals who face a probability of contracting a specific disease sometime in the future fall into a limbo somewhere between health and illness. Perhaps, in our alphabet soup world, they will become a new risk category called PPD – possibly, potentially diseased – or DIW – diseased in waiting. These PPDs or DIWs could range on a low-to-high risk continuum depending on the probability estimate attached to their acquiring the predicted disease and on the number of years this is expected to take.

Detecting potentially deleterious genes without providing amelioration poses serious questions for our social institutions – particularly those of law and medicine. Our present medical and legal systems are not designed to deal with the rights, privileges, obligations (or reduction of them) attaching to members of the PPD category.

The medical profession serves as the legitimator of illness or health status and social control agent. For example, the 'doctor's note' has many functions. If it states that you are healthy, it is used as the passport to employment. An equivalent note stating that you are sick allows exit from work, triggering receipt of sick benefits and disability claims. Predictive medicine now adds confusing elements into the existing ways of assigning health status. The distinction between probability and prediction is not always being made. Furthermore, the validity and reliability of the predictions are sometimes questionable. Health care providers, clients, family, schools, employers, the government and private insurers will be operating within a 'new world order' – probably as unstable as the political one.

What training should medical schools and refresher courses provide in probability based clinical applications and their social and ethical implications? As the division between health and illness is blurred will society's concept of the physician as well as the role of physician also change? What protection should the newly vulnerable have? Could the PPDs socially and legally maintain the status of being healthy without question marks, caveats and limitations being placed on this status?

Self/other interrelations: changes in social construction
The 'newly knowable' information about genetic makeup not only blurs the line between health and illness, but also blurs the line between normal variation and pathology. Thus, the new social norms arising from the clinical applications of recombinant DNA technology will affect how people see themselves, as well as how others see them.

No longer will people be able to say, 'What you see is what you get.' People's identity will change over time as more genes are identified, genetic screening tests developed and treatments for defects provided.

> Perhaps much of what we are looking at, when defined as pathology (particularly for multifactorial diseases), will be due to the same genes that determine normal variation when present as other alleles or in single rather than double dose. If so, the distinction between human and medical genetics becomes even more blurred, because in medical genetics we are looking at extremes but, by definition, much of the time we are looking at the same genes that determine normal variation.
> (Williamson 1990 p. 195)

A whole new vocabulary pertaining to individuals' genetic makeup is likely to enter the vernacular, just as ultrasound and amniocentesis have become household words for those of reproductive age. We will be talking about 'alleles' (genes at a locus on a chromosome that differ in their DNA sequences), 'polymorphic alleles' (loci at which at least 2 per cent of the population carry a variant allele), being 'homozygous' (having the same allele at a specific locus on both chromosomes), being 'heterozygous' (having a different allele at a specific locus on each chromosome), and 'degree of expressivity or penetration' (variations in age of onset and in severity of clinical manifestations, if any). Individuals will begin to ask whether some of their alleles are deleterious, part of normal variation, or beneficial. What criteria do you use to characterize yourself as a normal healthy person? Do you keep a score card weighing positive alleles against negative ones?

The concept of genetic responsibility may also alter the sense of self. Does it include the obligation to reveal knowledge about one's genetic makeup to partners, nuclear family and extended kinship and future generations? Will a new ethos based on the concept of an 'interdependent self' be developed, at least with respect to our genetic makeup. Markus and Kitayama (1991) found differences in the way members of Western cultures and members of Eastern cultures view themselves. In the West, the independent self based on individual autonomy is highly valued. In the East, the self includes significant others (interdependent self). This interest in the needs of others with whom one has close relationships, for example, a spouse, a parent, or child, is not considered separate from the self but an integral part of the self. In Western cultures, paradoxically, a shift to a concept of an interdependent self in relation to 'ownership' of genetic information may emerge as an ethical model at the very same time that society is leaning toward a reductionist model of 'humanhood' based on genetic identity. This duality is also seen in the intensive search for more sophisticated prenatal diagnostic and screening tests occurring concurrently with successful efforts to mainstream people with disabilities.

Most ethicists agree that only the individual concerned has the right to reveal personal genetic data and the right to determine who else should know. This right, however, is beginning to be qualified and may come under eventual attack, especially when treatments for some genetic defects are developed. Zimmerly (1990) states that an individual has the obligation to share the right of determining who should know strictly private personal genetic data with partners and other family members concerned.

The acceptance of an interdependent self as the norm for the sharing of private genetic information might lead to 'genetic cheating', a new form of deviance in conjugal relationships. The Catholic church now grants annulments when prior to the marriage one prospective partner lies or withholds crucial information from the other that might have influenced the decision to marry. In the future, would one basis for annulments (or divorces, in the case of other religions) include hiding genetic information or refusing to be tested if one partner knew that s/he might be at more than average risk?

Some of the same issues of responsibility – notifying partners and decisions to have children – arise in the case of an individual who tests HIV positive and are reflected in the laws relating to the spread of syphilis (Andrews and Jaeger 1991). When new medical technologies are available, categories of individuals often get transformed into new categories of potential clients. The medicalization of normal processes of birth and death, where intervention is not always beneficial is an example, and segments of society are fighting back with the return to midwifery and the design of 'living wills'. It is possible that the new genetic information will create a new health care category and a new stigmatized social category. This is particularly likely if the United States continues to emphasize individual responsibility rather than the interaction between the individual and the social and physical environment in its public health promotion campaigns.

The erosion of the norm of personal privacy

The norm of personal privacy is currently under attack. The norm is sanctified verbally, but its parameters are being redefined into a new entity not yet fully formed. When a long-standing norm is curtailed or circumscribed during period of rapid social change, the ensuing anomie frequently results in deleterious social consequences. The introduction of new technology is often the catalyst that sets off this cycle.

In the not too distant past, individuals could make themselves inaccessible if they wanted physical privacy or hide information about themselves if they wanted 'inner' privacy. This is no longer possible. People can seldom hide physically any more and increasingly, they cannot hide private information about themselves. Cellular phones, fax machines, phones in cars, planes and trains and telephone beepers can reach people almost anywhere, and computerized data banks hold tantalizing pieces of personal data that are too often insufficiently protected. Leaks of supposedly protected information have become all too common, and additional sensitive material will be discovered inadvertently as automated methods of genetic testing are improved.

In the not too distant future, a time-bomb conception of tomorrow may supersede present conceptions of time and distort previously accepted priorities of everyday life. PPDs will await the 'double whammy'of a time-bomb indicating leaks of their purportedly 'damaged' statuses combined with a time-bomb indicating the arrival of their possibly, potential diseases. If the norm of personal privacy is eroded, other socially acceptable protective mechanisms will evolve. But in the meantime, individuals may use deviant means such as lying and tampering with computer data to protect themselves from the release of genetic information that could be used to their detriment. In a society full of time bombs, social bonds previously internalized by members of the society may fray. 'As our diagnostic technology becomes more sophisticated there will be many [other] examples of sensitive information being acquired by chance as part of a diagnostic procedure.' (Weatherall 1991 p. 29).

Even when sensitive information is not acquired by chance, individuals often feel as though they have to release private information 'voluntarily' in order to obtain a job, life assurance, or health insurance (Gostin 1991). Furthermore, public health policy concerns itself with the community, rather than the individual, and tends to support norms emphasizing the rights of the group.

This social climate has been spawned by two powerful revolutions – the information systems revolution and the biomedical revolution. Their intersection has resulted in the development of parallel sets of norms, one set protecting privacy of personal information and another protecting the citizen's right of access to public information

(Zimmerly 1990). The boundaries between the two will be increasingly difficult to define clearly.

In order to clarify the boundary between these two types of rights with respect to genetic information, Zimmerly distinguishes between 'strictly private personal genetic data' describing a particular person which nobody is entitled to reveal, and 'publicly accessible personal genetic data' information about the *generally valid principle* describing the relationship between genes and their expressions (nobody is entitled to withhold this). But Zimmerly gives himself an important exception that equally blurs the distinction.

> It is quite obvious that every human being has a *moral right* to preserve his/her genetic privacy, at least to the same extent as he/she has the right to preserve his/her *social* privacy. However, it is equally obvious that nobody should be entitled to claim genetic privacy if somebody else, and/or a higher value, would be seriously endangered by it. On the basis of this we already see that genetic privacy is not an unconditionally defendable 'categoric' good.
>
> (Zimmerly 1990 p. 96)

If society accepts that individuals have the obligation to reveal genetic information when concealment could potentially harm others – knowing that they carry a susceptibility-conferring gene or disease-causing gene – what happens to the protection of 'strictly private genetic data'? While the international data bank for the scientific community is designed for publicly accessible data, the technological ability to store and access data, combined with a social mandate tilted toward the public good rather than individual privacy, may shift and widen the definition of publicly accessible genetic information.

Concern for the 'right of genetic privacy' has been expressed in many countries, and they have handled the issues in slightly different ways. For example, Germany has invoked constitutional principles which lead to a 'right of informational self-determination', while the United States has applied the principles of medical ethics to genetic screening (Zimmerly 1990). While these intents are noble, the reality is that invasion of personal privacy is becoming subtly acceptable.

For example, ultrasound is used routinely, even though professional guidelines do not recommend its universal use (Public Health Service 1984). Because it is considered to be routine rather than prenatal diagnosis, informed consent is not required (Lippman 1991). Furthermore, the House of Representatives recently passed a bill to restore federal funding for human foetal tissue research. To pacify opponents of such research, the bill includes a provision requiring women who are willing to donate foetal material for research to state in writing that they did not plan an abortion in order to donate foetal tissue. Researchers are required to keep the certifications in their files, which would be available for audit by state and federal officials. This bill makes no provision for protecting confidentiality, does not state whose property these certifications become, or require that the woman be informed of the conditions under which these statements will be used or stored (Kearny *et al.* 1991). The erosion of the right to privacy in cases not clearly earmarked as being ethically sensitive is likely to continue.

CONCLUSION

The potentially vulnerable and potentially sick are created when diagnostic techniques can predict future diseases with less than perfect certainty. The potentially stigmatized are created when this information is distorted and misused. All three categories already exist, but a growing number of individuals will fall into the first two categories and, perhaps, the third. When a majority, or even a substantial minority, of individuals fall into these categories, there will be a change in the way society perceives its members, defines their role obligations and structures their rights. Why have these issues been neglected? When they have been raised, why have they been, more often than not, treated as 'details' to be worked out?

Control over nature has been a dominant theme in American culture. Outer space (space missions) and inner space (probing the secrets of DNA) provide new and fertile fields. Moreover, overconfidence in the power of technology to solve problems is still endemic, despite increased opposition and counter trends (e.g. natural childbirth, death with dignity). Too frequently, prediction outstrips performance whether we are referring to a 'smart bomb' for a 'clean war', a bionic man with an artificial heart or a reduction in genetic disease and parental distress by carrier screening and prenatal diagnosis (Frets *et al.* 1991; Hodgkinson *et al.* 1990; Preston 1994). Limited performance is often transformed into a success story by political and professional rhetoric and amply portrayed in the media (Preston 1994). Nay-sayers are portrayed as Luddites mired in a nostalgic longing for an earlier, better time that never really existed.

Economics also plays a role in the social construction of the HGP. Gentech companies launched with venture capital have a vested interest in promoting the benign and optimistic image of applied human genetics, and employers, insurance companies and the government, all facing rapidly rising medical costs, grab at a 'technological fix' to solve their fiscal difficulties.

Those most worried about the rapid incorporation of genetic technology are found among academics, feminists and right-to-life advocates. Their concerns are so diverse that they are not likely to unite into an effective opposition. Furthermore, apprehensions regarding the impact on society's values, norms and institutions appear minor and esoteric compared to the alleviation of human suffering held out as the objective. Therefore, it is not at all surprising that the arguments against funding a large HGI are almost always answered by promising to prevent the *misuse* of an advance that is viewed as a tremendous benefit when used properly. Some scientists believe that their role is to do 'pure research', a value free endeavour, and distance themselves from any responsibility of society to curb the abuse of applied genetic technology. This function, they argue, belongs to the domain of lawyers, ethicists and physicians.

But misuse of technology and overselling benefits are not the only concerns. There are larger social ramifications. Probability produces uncertainty, which is disturbing to a society educated to think in absolutes. Hence, actuarial probability tends to be converted into case-by-case prediction at an individual level. Once a risk is quantified and labelled, it tends to be elided into a certainty. The label then attaches a new social and medical status to the individual, who becomes a member of a socially created category of people. This new label, whether it is 'mentally retarded' or 'high-risk', influences the way this category of people is treated irrespective of the uncertainties involved in the diagnosis or the number of false positives or false negatives involved.

More importantly, the process generates socially constructed 'at risk' categories and 'needs for technical solutions' (Lippman 1991). Nowhere can this be more clearly seen than in the field of applied human genetics. American society seems to be treading the path from medicalization to geneticization of social issues (Duster 1990; Lippman 1991).

REFERENCES

Anderson, C. (1991), 'Privacy bill vetoed', *Nature*, CCCLIII, p. 687
Andrews, L. and Jaeger, A. (1991), 'Confidentiality of genetic information in the workplace', *American Journal of Law and Medicine*, XVII, pp. 75–108

Beaudet, A. L. (1990), 'Invited editorial: carrier screening for cystic fibrosis', *American Journal of Human Genetics*, XLVII, pp. 603–5

Beckwith, Jon (1991) 'The Human Genome Initiative: genetics' lightning rod', *American Journal of Law and Medicine*, XVII, pp. 6–7

Brenner, S. (1990), 'Discussion', *Human Genetic Information: Science, Law and Ethics*, Ciba Foundation symposium 149, Wiley, Chichester, p. 93

Bobrow, M. and Manners, E. (1994), 'The social consequences of advances in the clinical applications of genetics', Chapter 2 This volume

Duster, T. (1990), *Backdoor to Eugenics*, Routledge, London

European Science Foundation (1991), *Report on Genome Research*, p. 11

Frets, P. C., Duivenboorden, H. J., Yerhage, F., Pers-Romeyn, E. M. T. and Niermeijer M. F. (1991), 'Analysis of problems in making the reproductive decision after genetic counselling', *Journal of Medical Genetics*, XXVIII, pp. 552–8

Friedmann, T. (1989), 'Progress toward human gene therapy', *Science*, CCXLIV, pp. 1275–81

——— (1990), 'Opinion: The Human Genome Project, some implications of extensive "reverse genetic" medicine', *American Journal of Human Genetics*, XLVI, pp. 407–14

Good, M. (1991), 'The political economy of hope: societal implications of the practice of oncology', paper presented at the Fulbright International Colloquium: The Social Consequences of Life and Death Under High Technology Medicine, 14–16 December 1991, Burnham, England

Gostin, L. (1991), 'Genetic discussion: the use of genetically based diagnostic and prognostic tests by employers and insurers', *American Journal of Law and Medicine*, XVII, pp. 109–44

Hodgkinson, K. A., Kerzin-Storar, L., Watters, E. A. and Harris, R. (1990), 'Adult polycystic kidney disease: knowledge, experience, and attitudes to prenatal diagnosis', *Journal of Medical Genetics*, XXVII, pp. 552–8

Holtzman, N. (1989), *Proceed with Caution: Predicting Genetic Risks in the Recombinant DNA Era*, Johns Hopkins University Press

Hurst, M. and Summey, P. (1984), 'Childbirth and social class: the case of cesarean delivery', *Social Science and Medicine*, XVIII, pp. 621–31

Jonas, H. (1985), 'Ethics and biogenetic art', *Social Research*, LII, pp. 491–504

Kearny, W., Vawter, D. and Gervais, K., (1991), 'Foetal tissue research and the misread compromise', *Hastings Center Report*, XXI, pp. 7–12

Kenen, R. (1994), 'Women and Risk', in F. Huttner, (ed.), *Our Vision and Values: Women Shaping the Twenty First Century*, Greenwood/Praeger, New York

Kenen, R. and Schmidt, R. (1978), 'Stigmatization of carrier status: social implications of heterozygote genetic screening programs', *American Journal of Public Health*, November, pp. 1116–20

Lippman, A. (1991), 'Prenatal genetic testing and screening: Constructing needs and reinforcing inequalities', *American Journal of Law and Medicine*, XVII, pp. 15–50

Lock, M. (1994), 'Contests with death: ideologies of nationalism and internationalism in Japan', Chapter 11 this volume

Markus, H. and Kitayama, S. (1991), 'Culture and the self: implications for cognition, emotion and motivation', *Psychological Review*, XCVIII, pp. 224–53

National Center for Human Genome Research, National Institutes for Health (no date), *The Human Genome Project: New Tools for Tomorrow's Health Research* (pamphlet)

—— (1991), *The Ethical, Legal and Social Implications of Human Genome Research: Preparing for the Responsible Use of New Genetic Knowledge* (executive summary)

Nelkin, D. and Tancredi, L. (1989), *Dangerous Diagnosis: The Social Power of Biological Information*, Basic Books, New York

Nossal, G. J. V. (1990), Introduction, *Human Genetic Information: Science, Law and Ethics*, Ciba Foundation symposium 149, Wiley, Chichester, pp. 1- 5

Preston, T. (1994), 'The social consequences of the development of the artificial-heart', Chapter 7, this volume

Public Health Service, US Department of Health and Human Services (1984), *Consensus Development Conference: Diagnostic Ultrasound Imaging in Pregnancy*, 11 (National Institutes of Health, Publication No. 167)

Shy, K. K., Luthy, D., Bennet, F. *et al.* (1990), 'Effects of electronic foetal- heart-rate monitoring', *The New England Journal of Medicine*, cccxxii, pp. 588–98

Strathern, M. (1994), 'Displacing knowledge: technology and its consequences for kinship', Chapter 5 this volume

Weatherall, D. (1991), 'Manipulating human nature', *SPA*, August pp. 25–30

Williamson, R. (1990), 'Discussion', *Human Genetic Information: Science, Law and Ethics*, Ciba Foundation symposium 149, Wiley, Chichester, pp. 32–3

Zimmerly, W. C. (1990), 'Who has the right to know the genetic constitution of a particular person?', *Human Genetic Information: Science, Law and Ethics*, Ciba Foundation symposium 149, Wiley, Chichester, pp. 93–102

5

Displacing knowledge: technology and its consequences for kinship

MARILYN STRATHERN

Referring to American ideas, David Schneider (1968 p. 23) once observed that kinship is whatever the biogenetic relationship is. 'If science discovers new facts about biogenetic relationship, then that is what kinship is and was all along, although it may not have been known at the time.' There are many other ways of defining kin persons, but no way of conceptualising a biogenetic tie between persons that does not presuppose it as a kinship tie. Schneider was writing in the 1960s. In the intervening years, developments in reproductive medicine have made the biogenetic basis of human relationships visible to an unprecedented degree. Does Schneider's statement also stand as a prediction? Are we uncovering new facts about kinship?

Anthropologists would have no difficulty in offering a general prediction. Given their relational view of the world, they might be expected to point out that the reproduction of human beings is also the reproduction of social relationships. What would they mean? There is the question of who is involved: high technology medicine has introduced new actors into the process of procreation – such as the assisting clinician, gamete donor or so-called surrogate mother.[1] There are bound to be consequences for relationships based on procreation. And there is also the question of how procreation occurs: the new actors contribute to a field of what might indeed be called new facts.

These are facts about ways in which procreation may be facilitated and what is entailed in the process. If a fact is new, the implication is that it adds to what already exists. It is this implication that leads me to hazard a specific prediction. The prediction is framed by the analytical assumption that cultural analysis is always after the event. What is presented as extrapolation into the future, then, is commentary on current practices. There are two parts to the extrapolation. First, if Schneider's statement belonged to a time when kinship was an axiomatic component of family life, then we might be looking forward to their separation. 'Kinship' relations could acquire a new autonomy apart from the family as an institution. Second, insofar as procreation (the process of conception and birth) were once regarded as an axiomatic component of reproduction (which refers both to the biological process of producing new children and to the perpetuation of aspects of personal identity over time), then we can also expect these to diverge. Personal 'identity' could become understood in terms of genetic substance rather than kin relationship. The outcome would be *a simultaneous emphasis and de-emphasis on relationships as such.* A field of kin relations would partially displace the family as the arena in which people worked out the implications of new procreative practices. At the same time, a genetic basis for personal identity would partially displace the evidence kinship once provided. 'Technology' will have aided both outcomes.

Insofar as the biogenetic basis of kin relations becomes more evident, then it would seem that the more we know, the more visible such kinship will be as a domain of relationships in its own right. Schneider's dictum would seem to hold. Yet were kin relationships to cease to occupy a foundational place in the way people think about other areas of life, including the origins of personal identity, it would cease to be kinship as we have known it. Why might techniques developed for medical ends, especially those that remedy or bypass impaired fertility, have such consequences? In foreshadowing my answer, I bring in a central concern of this chapter.

Schneider's observation was, in the first instance, an observation about *knowledge:* how we make facts known. Cultural life is lived through the constant displacement of knowledge. There is nothing new here. We move between contexts, draw analogies, forget this in order to concentrate on that, extend our vision and, above all, return to previous positions again. Often what is displaced is only over the horizon, there to be recovered. But there is a special effect that arises from the desire to make known or explicit facts otherwise assumed to be foundational. The displacement effect of uncovering assumptions, of making the implicit explicit, sets off an irreversible process. The implicit can never be recovered, and there is no return to old assumptions – displacement becomes radical.

Developments in reproductive medicine do not just comprise new procedures; they also embody new knowledge. In redefining the conditions under which it is possible to live or die, reproductive technology puts people in the position of making new kinds of choice in the context of new kinds of information (for example Rapp 1989). The ramifications of ethical and social consequences seem endless. What a student of culture might add is that exploring the implications of such innovation is not simply a matter of showing an ever-increasing range of information that adds to what is previously known and thus opens up fresh avenues. We shall also be witnessing a substitutive effect, the way avenues are also closed off. And that is because new knowledge always works on old. There is no vacuum in people's practices and habits of thought; there are only existing practices and habits of thought on which the new will work. In some cases, old practices lie in wait, as I have said, with their questions and doubts. In other cases displacement may be radical: if new knowledge takes away old assumptions, it will have put new assumptions in their place.

EURO-AMERICAN KINSHIP

The fact that kinship is whatever the biogenetic relationship is sounds self-evident. Indeed, it is one of the 'facts of life' Euro-Americans take for granted. Whoever acts the part of parent, a biogenetic tie with genitor or genetrix in and of itself also indicates parenthood. Presumably that is what 'parent' would indicate in zoological terminology where a social relationship is not at issue. Such, for example, is how I would understand Clifford Grobstein's reference to kinship. This former embryologist wishes to draw attention to the linkages between generations effected through the transmission of genetic material; the outcome, he says, is a 'hereditary web . . . [and] within the web there are kin relationships among members of a generation and also between succeeding generations' (1990 p. 20).

Schneider argues that it is as a set of natural facts that such ties are held to lie at the heart of the social relationships in which human beings also engage: 'kinship is defined as biogenetic' (1968 p. 23). When Grobstein uses 'kinship' in a biogenetic sense, and when Americans use 'biogenetics' in a kinship sense, perhaps each thereby adds to their factual understanding of the world. Yet for an anthropologist, Schneider's statement is factual in a special sense. Anthropological knowledge transposes the facticity at stake, from a domain of natural facts to a domain of cultural ones. The full sentence reads: '[i]n American cultural conception, kinship is defined as biogenetic' (1968 p. 23, my emphasis).

Here is an example of the displacement effect of knowledge. As soon as one has realised that a fact is also a cultural artefact,[2] displacement takes effect. The anthropologist can always return to the natural facticity implied in the idea of biogenetic kinship, as becomes someone acting with reference to their own culture. But the position can no longer be assumed axiomatically.[3] Anyone interested in crosscultural comparison would recognise the statement about biogenetic kinship as culturally charged. Although everywhere there are special social arrangements attendant on the production and rearing of children, it is not the case that everywhere the core of ties so established between kin are ultimately understood as having their origins in procreation. Ties of substance and the nature of bodily constitution may be determined by non-procreative factors such as nurture, the intervention of ancestral spirits or even the nature of the land where one is (to be) buried: bio- without the genetics, and created but not necessarily procreated.

There are, of course, many dimensions to Euro-American relations of kinship beyond those afforded by procreation. Examples abound in Finch's (1989) recent study of family obligations in England. There are diverse rationales for the relationships that arise in the course of family life, and a diversity of rationales exists everywhere. The concept of a 'blood tie' or of persons being of 'one's own flesh and blood' refers simply to the foundation of intimate relationships in natural processes. Yet it is not the case world-wide that the foundation of relationships is held to rest in such biogenetic facts. That is a distinctively Euro-American rendition. And while 'flesh and blood' might be a symbol, it is a symbol for what Euro-Americans take to be literally true: that those joined by substance are kin, and it is the act of procreation that accomplishes the joining.[4] The circumstances of conception and birth that make the child also make it a kinship entity, and when Euro-Americans think of people reproducing themselves, they mean first and foremost through procreation.[5] In this sense, procreation is at the core of reproduction.

There is much scope here for empirical enquiry and the investigation of concrete cases; indeed we know lamentably little about how Euro-Americans regularly formulate such issues. This chapter cannot remedy that deficit. But it can draw attention to the concreteness of the forms that Euro-American knowledge takes, and to the cultural repertoire that is available for people to think with however they apply it to specific circumstances. For while one cannot predict future cultural configurations, one can reflect on the place that existing concepts hold in present-day cultural practice. Thus, abstract as it might sound, I take the concept of a 'natural fact' as foundational to Euro-American perceptions of the primordial base to human relations. In the same way, the family has certain characteristics that mark it off by cultural definition from other institutions of modern society. Although such ideas and concepts may appear abstract by contrast with what people do or think in specific circumstances, as cultural reference points they are decidedly concrete by contrast with the abstract potential of everything that may get done or thought, and open to empirical enquiry.

Data in the following sections derive from a range of sources, including contemporary debates surrounding the Human Fertilisation and Embryology Act 1990, as they have been reported in the press or filtered through academic publications, and a preliminary investigation of the impact of reproductive technology on the representation of kinship.[6] The past tense will refer to the mid-century cultural milieu of which Schneider was writing.

Let me briefly explain that ugly term 'Euro-American'. I need an epithet to highlight the cultural specificity of the kinship system that is most immediately affected by the new reproductive technologies, although they are by no means confined to it.[7] The system is found across North America and Northern Europe, but is not tied to locale, though it may be tied to class or to the late-twentieth-century 'classlessness' or apparent cosmopolitanism afforded by communications technology. It also once contributed to a larger world view that saw social relationships as built up after the facts of nature. I use the past tense because it is that foundationalism that is now under challenge. If one of the distinctive characteristics of this system was the value placed on procreation and thus on parentage (see Schneider 1984; Bloch 1987) in the definition of kin relations, it is a system likely to be responsive to changes in procreative practice.

Historically speaking, the world view that took natural facts as a domain for scientific investigation is, of course, the world view that promoted certain conditions for medical development (treating the human body as a system) and that provided kinship with a symbolic basis in nature. Kinship was seen to be what people did with the natural circumstances of birth. The idea that kin relations were grounded in a domain of natural facts at once gave the relationships an axiomatic facticity *and* rendered them contingent on the natural facts themselves and thus on what could be known about them. Hence natural facts could be treated in their own right – as in techniques to assist conception – and without reference to social relations; but the reverse was not true, for any definition of parent-child or sibling relations had to take the natural facts into account.

When I refer to Euro-American kinship ideas, I mean those based on such post-Enlightenment, modernist axioms. Nowadays they are disseminated through the communication network once the prerogative of the educated middle classes. They inhere in the discourse of most North European/American academics and professionals, and constitute a way of thinking about human relations and what society or culture does with them. The interesting question is what the products of this kinship system have done to themselves in enhancing procreative success. For sure, they will not reproduce the system that produced them.

KINSHIP AND THE DISPLACEMENT OF FAMILY

Insofar as reproductive medicine affords new ways of 'knowing' about kinship, and in so doing displaces old ones, the first displacement turns on how family members know themselves as kin. Among the concerns of both the Warnock (1985) and Glover (1989) Reports were people's apparent preoccupation with the future of the nuclear family. 'The family' is, of course, perennially under threat; indeed, one might begin worrying if it were not. In the meanwhile, there seems no reason why, as a domestic institution, the family should wither away. We may even expect family members to continue to see themselves as related through sexual and parental ties. When I refer to its displacement I do not mean that the family will disappear. I mean that there will be more to kinship than family life. One might think this has 'always been' the case. Extended family networks (see Wilson and Pahl 1988) have always been an extra-domestic dimension to family life. Yet these were formerly constituted in the way membership of the nuclear family was constituted, through the mechanics of procreation and marriage; it was just that relationships grew less direct the 'further out' kin reckoning extended. However variably relatives were treated, the fact of relationship remained grounded in those biogenetic and affinal suppositions. Closeness of biogenetic identity symbolised degrees of closeness between kin.

As a consequence, 'kinship' as a network of more or less close connections radiating out from the individual could always be separated from the family as an institution based on conjugal companionship and the rearing of children. But what gave Euro-American culture its modernist cast in this regard was that the core of the family was constituted in the procreative act of the conjugal pair in such a way that the child's biogenetic closeness to its parents endorsed the nurturing closeness of the conjugal couple. Though they were not born kin to each other, the child was born kin to both of them. The child they produced created a 'closeness' defined in the way familial and kinship relations overlapped.

The new actors associated with reproductive medicine create a field of relationships that does not overlap in any simple way with familial ones. It is not that the facts of procreation will necessarily take precedence over other grounds for creating a family, and indeed the procreative facts have never been the only 'natural' facts to which family members may appeal.[8] But when there were other reasons, these were often simply supplemental to the facts of procreation – the need to nurture a dependant, assist the development of a child – and caretaking roles could be dispersed among several persons. In some of the current facilities offered by assisted conception, it is the range of those involved *in procreation itself* that has become dispersed. The child is 'produced' by the couple who want it, but the kinship is dispersed. What was once a symbol for 'closeness' in familial relations may now bring in persons 'distant' to one another.[9] Dispersed kinship is constituted in dispersed conception, for this includes those who 'produce' the child with assistance as well as those who 'assist'. As a consequence, there thus exists a field of procreators whose relationship to one another and to the product of conception are contained in the act of conception itself and not in the family as such.

Indeed, the whole weight of legislative intervention in Britain has been to ensure that 'the family' is protected from interference by third parties, even as gamete donors may be protected from family claims being made on them.[10] Everything, as is also true of this kinship system,[11] is further qualified by reference to what people want. Thus the whole issue of donor anonymity (in DI) and what the donor 'wants' is compromised by what is thought good for the child, which in turn anticipates what the child might 'want' in the future. Such qualifications may lead to the family being seen as the beneficiary of assistance received from persons whose role is defined strictly in relation to the act of procreation. Such protection thereby locates (aspects of) the procreative process 'outside' the family.

All a family may be said to be doing is repairing bits and pieces of its own functioning and thus strengthening its sense of itself. It may either endorse the importance of procreation (see note 9) in seeking the outside assistance to remedy procreative impairment, or fall back on a non-procreative definition of familial ties. It is no paradox, then, that 'the family' seems as vigorous a concept as ever.

To disperse procreation, however, is to displace its place in the ways Euro-Americans think about the family. That in terms of the total population only a few are ever involved directly in such procedures is a triviality; these ways of thinking are now available to everyone. What is interesting, then, is that no-one denies that being an actor in the process of conception establishes a relationship. The kind of legal recognition she receives is another matter, but the 'surrogate' mother is already a surrogate 'mother'. The personal identity of the anonymous semen donor may be unknown, but he is still the biological 'father'. Couples can even be referred to as relinquishing 'genetic parenthood' (King's Fund Centre 1991). If mothers, fathers and parents are still kin, then procreation continues to produce kinship.

And it is as a consequence that one may expect a 'new kinship' as well as new family forms to flourish. The idea of dispersed conception does not have to remain tied to the technological procedures necessary for ova extraction or the tendency to medicalise donor insemination. Indeed, we 'already know' the varieties of domestic arrangements that characterise late-twentieth-century ideas of family life – whether a consequence of divorce and remarriage or the expression of diverse sexual preferences or a politicisation of domestic style itself. But making visible the detachment of the procreative act from the way the family produces a child adds new possibilities to the conceptualisation of intimacy in relationships. However minimal the role of those involved, dispersed conception may provide a model for relations that can take on a kinship character even where they cannot take on a family one.

Should we then go back to the Enlightenment origins of the modernist world view to which the Euro-American kinship system of much of the twentieth century has belonged? Will kinship as the basis for family life come to seem a remote historical interlude? Shall we undo the process of domestification that produced the nuclear family as the middle class have known it for as long as they too have existed (see Davidoff and Hall 1987)? Are we about to return to some pre-industrial separation of family from (kinship) 'connection'?

While it is entertaining to imagine a return to older practices, the thought is no more than that. What established the naturalness of family life in the industrial world was the naturalness of the biological functions it was seen to carry out. This is what made family members kin to one another. And the kinship system I have been describing was coterminous with an understanding of nature as biology. Euro-Americans came to know the procreative process as a biological fact, and they came to know that procreation creates a kinship that was founded first and foremost in biogenetic relationships. Go back to the non-familial kin 'connections' of the eighteenth century and you have gone back to a different and pre-Darwinian apprehension of nature itself (see Strathern 1992, Chapter 3). Subsequent knowledge will have made return impossible.

PROCREATION AND THE DISPLACEMENT OF REPRODUCTION

One might envisage kinship acquiring new prominence. A cultural paradox is nonetheless produced by the fact that 'more' kinship does not necessarily lead to 'more' relatives. Thus while the kinship field now includes a miscellany of actors assembled for the purposes of procreation, not all biogenetic relationships may be activated as social ones. Yet the social activation of relationships is central to what we may think of as reproduction.

Euro-American kinship always made it possible for one to be related without activating the relationship. (One may know one has a father, but not who he is; or one may know who he is, but not act like his child.) When a kin relationship is activated, it is of course acted upon either because what was always known provides the basis for social interaction (as in the way kin select those they keep up with) or else because what was not before known becomes so (and the person with the knowledge has to act on it in some way, even if only to resolve not do anything more with the knowledge). However, the facts of procreation that establish kinship refer to a physical process that, beyond telling us that the act also creates a relationship between creator/created, is neutral as to the nature of that relationship.

Procreation creates, then, but is such a creation also 'reproduction'? I seize on the difference of terms to describe the second displacement effect of biogenetic knowledge. Reproduction commonly means to bring into existence something that already exists in another form. The form may be duplicated (as in making a copy), regenerated (as in making anew), in a symbolic relationship to the original (as in representing it) or is recalled (as in bringing it to the memory or imagination). As biology is understood by the lay person, reproduction appears as the process by which an original plant or animal produces individuals similar to itself. Euro-American understandings of the similarities involved in human reproduction are, of course, not at all neutral as to the nature of relationship at issue. A relationship is thought to inhere in a continuity of (personal) identity.

Now that implies, I think, that reproduction cannot occur in the absence of a certain kind of knowledge: that is, knowledge about the identity of others. While it is possible to think of the anonymous semen donor (say) as the unknown biological father of the child, it would be culturally stretching the point to think of that donor as engaged in an act of reproduction. The Euro-American idea of human reproduction trails the supposition that in some sense one recreates (part of) oneself. That part must be 'known' or 'seen' in another specific person to be effective.

In this sense, procreation was once a symbol of reproductive continuity. We can appreciate the cultural force of all those idioms of possession which indicate the desire to transmit aspects of oneself – and if not body parts then property or way of life – to the future.[12]

The very idea of continuity between generations is contained in the idea of a downward flow of characteristics. The reverse lies in the desire to trace origins, establish roots, claim inheritance. But what used to be a condition of being in the world, that a person was the repository of a whole mix of elements in the course of transmission, and thus the object of another (specific) person's reproduction, is rendered contingent in the possibilities offered by the new technology.

The technological interventions that separate kinship from family also separate procreation from reproduction. By contrast with other remedies for childlessness such as adoption, couples may seek medical procedures, such as in-vitro fertilisation, precisely in order to be able to reproduce as much of themselves as possible. Yet the technologies are, so to speak, indifferent to the social origins of egg and sperm, the persons from whom they come, even to where gestation takes place. When initial treatments fail, others may be suggested, and intending parents may thus be led into relocating what it is of themselves they reproduce. If it is finally the intention or desire to have a child which remains intact, then that is what the child 'reproduces'. So in becoming a means to fulfil such a desire, procreation itself ceases to be the crucial reproductive moment.[13] We might see that moment instead as the acting out of intention or desire. In the case of anonymous gamete onation, the identity of the procreative material is screened out of the parent(s)' reproductive endeavour; and as far as the donors are concerned, the efficacy of their procreative act need have no consequences for their reproduction.[14] I do not mean that identity necessarily remains concealed (see Snowden and Mitchell 1983, apropos DI). I mean that, *whether or not* people know, there is a sense in which the knowledge becomes culturally ancillary. From the point of view of the commissioning parents, the identity of donor parties may be deliberately held at bay or be regarded as intrusive to the act of reproduction, that is, to the fulfilment of a person in becoming a parent. (The breach proves the rule. Where a known person is sought out, as can be the case in the donation of ova, the identity of the donor may on the contrary be important in duplicating the identity of the intending parent(s): here procreative identity does have reproductive implications.) From the point of view of the donors, it is interesting to consider the Report of the King's Fund Centre Counselling Committee (1991)[15] concerning guidelines for the regulation of infertility treatment. The Committee considered counselling to be essential for donors as well as recipients of gametes, and the issues they list include the possibility of the donor's own 'childlessness'. One infers that donors might be childless not because their procreative material was infertile but because it did not lead to 'their' child being born. In short, the procreative act did not lead to reproduction.

Knowledge about biological process adds a further element. I refer here to popular renditions of biology,[16] and to 'knowledge' not in respect of the object known (which may according to other evidence be accurate or inaccurate) but with respect to the way such objects are incorporated as foundational assumptions. Euro-Americans have learnt that the essential copying function in the creating of new persons is carried out by 'the genes'.

People may be aware that there are many other aspects of coming into being, including the triggering mechanisms which make the genetic code efficacious, nurture, the environment of the gestatory vessel, and so forth. It is also understood that genes express themselves in varied ways, and that 'having' a gene for a characteristic does not guarantee that the characteristic will show itself. But it is 'known' that without the genetic disposition for that characteristic, no amount of external influence will produce it. So genes are thought of as providing a range of potentials, some of which will actualise. Actualised or not,[17] all of them contribute to a person's identity.

Now Euro-Americans also 'know' the consequence: that persons are thereby programmed for life.[18] Once you have them, it does not in this sense make any difference where the genes are from. They are essential for procreation (in the absence of genetic instruction there is no organism), and procreation is equally essential for them (without an organism there are no genes). But from the point of view of the person who is procreated, 'reproduction' need not come into the picture at all. A person can be procreated without at the same time reproducing *other persons.*

I make this statement on the grounds of late-twentieth-century cultural logic: the origin and social identity of genetic material is not relevant to its efficacy. At the same time, rapidly increasing knowledge about the complexity of genetic make-up displaces any simple reckoning of traits being passed down through family lines. There always was a kind of gradation in traditional kinship beliefs, an assumption that one was likely to reproduce more of the characteristics that showed in one's parents than (say) showed in one's grandparents. While it was always possible to 'see' even remote relatives 'in' this or that child, by and large persons 'took after' their mother or father. If this primitive knowledge of the inheritance of characteristics is being displaced by knowledge about genetic mapping, then the simple idea that one person passed on a characteristic to another, like a piece of property, may become displaced by a sense of the complex way in which elements combine.

Now from the point of view of an individual person, the consequences of genetic endowment are all one way. How you manifest things may reveal the constitution of the parent from whom you inherited, but knowledge of this process affects neither their constitution nor yours. And while in personal/social terms it may matter considerably to individuals to know who their genetic parents are, the body retains its genetic composition independently of this knowledge. You do not need to know the identity of your parents in order to fall ill from this or that genetic disorder inherited from them.

This re-introduces the cultural paradox. The more knowledge Euro-Americans have of the likelihood of disorders being transmitted, and the ever-increasing accuracy with which genetic components can be traced, the less necessary it becomes to know the identity of the parent. More kinship, fewer relatives! In the recent past the physical behaviour or symptoms that a parent or another kinsperson manifested yielded information about the possibility of such traits having been passed on. Since family histories were used to make inferences about genetic disposition, kinship genealogies were medically important for tracing the 'inheritance' of genetic defects.[19] Nowadays it is possible to imagine direct access to the genome itself. If '[T]here is no essential difference between reading the genes by a patient's description of their symptoms and family history *and reading them directly*' (Brenner

1991, p. 37, my emphasis) then all one need know is what one has. No difference for diagnosis may, of course, entail every difference for how to think about ancestry.

In the old vocabulary of blood ties, the connection of substance presumed to lie between persons acted as a reference point or symbol for the immutability of relationships. It was an implicit foundation on which they were built. As we have seen, however, finding out more information about the foundations does not necessarily lead to more information about the relationships. Explicitness has a displacement effect: one form of knowledge takes the place of another. Genetics is not only about blood ties, and thus about ancestry; it is also about the unique constellation of characteristics that make up individuals. In the former case, relations were evident as ties between specific persons; in the latter case, they contributed the components of the individual person's make-up. It would seem that the more we know about this constellation, the less we shall in fact need to know about the relationships. Perhaps, as Rabinow (1990) hints with reference to ethnic characteristics, individuals will in the future come to be seen as belonging to genetic 'populations' and 'sub-populations'.

Now that double possibility – that identity may *or* may not be located with reference to specific other persons – is already a part of Euro-American kinship thinking.[20] Consider what Birke *et al.* have pointed to as an obsession with genes in popular understandings of embryo development.

The obsession belongs, they suggest, to a biologically outmoded paradigm of development as mere unfolding. 'The belief that genes ... define us as individuals from the moment of conception' (1990, p. 67) has, they later say, no biological foundation: we should recognise such ideas for the ideological devices they are (1990, p. 73). The ideology is not, of course, free-floating. It is part of a constellation of ideas about human nature, and one which carries that double reference to identity. If knowledge of genetic inheritance ('heredity') adds to the ways of thinking about social inheritance, it both invokes relations with other persons (one's link with the past, one's ancestry) and invokes the individual (to whom inheritance exists as a resource or endowment). The same double inheres in Euro-American concepts of nurture, at once invoking others (one person is enfolded within the care of another) and invoking the single being who is the object of their care (nurture attends to the biological/social needs of the individual). Here the relationship between parent and child is paradigmatic. Between parent and child Euro-Americans see both a relation between persons *and* the tending of individual development – both the interpersonal tie and a need to provision the growing child. In the latter sense parents supply background, environment, the supports that will carry the child through life.[21] Hence the power of the genetic imagery. It, too, offers a double focus: what other persons make is the unique individual.[22]

The new knowledge of 'genetics' that is filtered through popular accounts of the genome might simply slot in here, adding to what we already know, were it not for other developments in the ordering of relationships. It is the new genetic knowledge in the context of new procreative possibilities that suggests radical displacement. The genome presents a different picture of hereditary material from the old notions of genes as bundles of traits. People now 'know' they are endowed not with traits but with the potential for them. Perhaps the significance of that potential will turn what once was a symbol for the immutables of human existence (genetic endowment) into a symbol for the open-endedness of possibilities (the realisation of potential) *that only the individual will manifest.*[23]

I suggest that because, in turn, of another Euro-American double, the human body. The body is thought to show both the imprint of other persons' care towards it and its (individual) potential for development from within.[24] In the second sense, the body is required to give evidence of its own state of being. So, however much categorisation is regarded as culturally derived or the dividing line as an arbitrary point in a process, the body must give evidence of whether or not it is alive or dead (see Lamb 1990), even as the embryo must present the signs of its own individuality (see Morgan and Lee 1991, Chapter 3). Here we may add that the new procreative arrangements do not attend to the commissioning parents' need for a child in some abstract or metaphoric sense: they are designed to produce a body that may become that child. Medicine must define the body first with respect to its internal viability, and only second with respect to the relations it embodies. This is the cultural context in which recent interest in the genome reveals the possibility of genetic mapping, documenting the individuality of the body that will be the object of the new parents' concerns.

So what about reproduction? New practices of reproduction would work out of an old kinship system that once endorsed the importance of knowing about body process. In its place, individual persons may well come to endorse their sense of autonomy in the self-referenial identity of a 'genetic profile'. In fact, in order to carry on thinking of the transmitters of disease as mothers and fathers, it might become necessary to screen off knowledge about one's genetic make-up from knowledge about one's hereditary origins. The continuity of inter-personal relationships could even depend on constructing one's inheritance in a discontinuous way! In the conduct of human inter-actions, might this, conversely, mean an emphasis away from genetic continuity (and genetic liability)?

Along the lines of such an extrapolation, might kin relationships come to be symbolised in a non-genetic mode? That is, the repro-duction of persons would be disassociated from the genetic impli-cations of procreation. Would it follow, then, that Euro-American kin constructs would come to seem more like those of (say) the people of Melanesia who never held a genetic theory of reproduction?

The immediate answer is that biological knowledge of bodily process would intervene. The non-procreational and non-genetic aspects of kin relations in Melanesia are (to the Euro-American anthropologist) recognisably kinship phenomena insofar as they attend to bodily con-stitution. Persons are related to persons through ties of substance and physical bonding even where such ties are not instigated through procreation. But in the Euro-American separation of procreation from reproduction, as I have hazarded in this section, it is likely that the substantial and bodily part of the person will continue to be regarded as constituted in his or her genetic make-up, and that is exactly what does not depend on a reproductive tie with the parent.

CONCLUSION

Kinship as Euro-Americans presently think of it does not 'go with' all these novel concepts with equal ease. In the separation of what I initially called kinship from family, I pointed to the potential nexus of relations (the 'new kinship') to which procreation gives rise making it no longer foundational for the family. But in the separation of procreation from reproduction, we find that the genetic tie that once symbolised the transmission of traits between persons, and thus the reproduction of one person in the person of another, now carries a new potential for individual identity. As part of the procreative rather than reproductive process, identity seems given in genetic endowment, and a relationship with another person is not necessary to that knowl-edge. Where, then, do we put 'kinship'?

In following through some of the conceptual consequences of the *new* reproductive technologies, I have given a kind of surrogate cultural analysis. Such extrapolation is the only form that a predictive cultural account can make; it must deal with what already exists. In so doing I have drawn attention to one significant dimension, and that is the place that knowledge holds in Euro-American kinship thinking.

That thinking was predicated on certain known facts about biology; and on the ways of knowing who a relative was. These two forms of knowledge replicate each other in that knowledge is seen to be after the fact. On the one hand it is about biological process, and the more we know about the process the more (it would seem) we know about what makes kinship. On the other hand, while the procreative act is constitutive of kinship in a biogenetic sense, making that knowledge explicit makes more not less evident the fact that the social relationship is contingent. What once underpinned Euro-American understandings of kinship now alters the place that social relationships held in ideas about primordial personal identity.

This has been a hypothetical exercise, although I have described nothing that does not already exist somewhere, for someone. The question is one of saliency. What I have not offered are generalisations about how people behave. If anything, I have been observing the way we may expect certain ideas to behave; they drive us as much as we draw on them. A brief example will serve as a conclusion.

In their commentary on the Human Fertilisation and Embryology Act, Morgan and Lee (1991, p. 165) report on part of the controversy over the need to know one's genetic ancestry. They quote an argument to the effect that, at least as far as adoptees are concerned, empirical evidence is simply lacking – we do not have the information to substantiate the claim that adoptees suffer an overwhelming urge to seek out their genitors. It is unclear, however, what exactly the empirical evidence would uncover. It might be very helpful to those involved in counselling or in interpreting the regulations surrounding adoption to know that most adoptees do not have an overwhelming desire to search for their identity. Yet the presumed 'search for identity' does not in the first place exist as a generalisation based on empirical fact. It exists as a comment on the foundations of human nature that presumes a modelling of social relationships into which adopted persons do not readily fit. The 'search for identity' is an idea, and it is the idea that drives.

Ideas drive insofar as one evokes another. There is no reason why in their daily lives adoptees or a child born to non-genetic parents should be preoccupied with a search for (biogenetic) identity any more than anyone else. But there is every reason why the idea should arise at those moments when they, or anyone else, think about the constitution of human nature in kinship, itself an idea. Thus Morgan and Lee introduce the topic of 'the need to know' in the context of 'genetic parentage', an issue that has much preoccupied those having to take a decision on the question of donor identity. It had to be dealt with, in the same way as the 'biological father' has to be dealt with in thinking about DI.

There are three aspects to such configurations of ideas. First, one idea leads to another: satisfying the need to know is felt to be part of being a complete person. But suppose it were thought desirable to uncouple such associations. Suppose, as in the argument the authors cite, it is urged that *instead* of focusing on the need to know one's genetic ancestry, one should concentrate on changing society's attitudes towards the importance of blood relationships. We observe, second, that the alternative works through replacing one piece of knowledge by another. After all, it is said, we know that need is socially induced.[25] Such knowledge is offered as a fresh insight, as new information that comes from an increasingly sophisticated awareness about the social construction of natural facts. But it does, of course, introduce a third effect, what I have called radical displacement. When knowledge is seen as 'new', it substitutes for old suppositions, and in adding may also subtract. We are invited to realise that an idea we thought was foundational (the need to know genetic ancestry) ought not to be so, since the inference is that if a need is socially induced, it ceases to be an inevitable fact of life.

The need to know that apparently drives the search for genetic identity is also crucial to the development of techniques to assist those who are childless through infertility. But what is learnt is often more than what we wanted to know. The results may be new grounds for medical uncertainty (see Price 1990). Or they may shift the cultural grounds on which knowledge itself is sought. Arguments about the individual's 'right to know' based on his/her rights to knowledge about him/herself are arguments for knowing about the individual rather than about the kinsperson. So while kinship in Euro-American thinking may be predicated on the facts of life, learning more about the facts of life will not necessarily tell us more about kinship.

Euro-American kinship was always about a kind of knowledge. Not just knowing who (who one's parents were as persons), but knowing how (the procreative process that created one as an individual). Knowledge in turn rested on another kind of foundational assumption: that one should act on what one knows. Until knowledge itself is displaced from the heart of this modelling of relationships, new knowledge will go on having consequences for it.

NOTES

1. The roles of these persons may all have existed before, and they are adjuncts to, rather than intrinsic to, the application of high technology techniques. But the point is that 'technology' gives them new visibility and legitimacy. Two examples are apposite. (1) Snowden's (1990 p. 101) expostulate during an interchange at the 1988 conference on philosophical ethics in reproductive medicine. Braude: [apropos DI] 'presumably the law must also apply to any child who wishes to know the identity of its father' [this would be impracticable if applied to everyone]; Snowden: 'But the state does not set up adultery centres!' [fertility clinics have introduced special practices]. (2) Lord Teviot's speech to the House of Lords (Embryology Bill, *Hansard*, 13 February 1990 col. 1307) apropos genetic parenthood on birth certificates:

   If we do not do anything to mark the certificates we are in effect abandoning any real claim that our birth certificates and birth registers show genetic relationships. In the past it was always an offence knowingly and wilfully to give wrong information to a registrar. It is one thing for an individual to give false information and to risk prosecution but quite another for a government to create a legal fiction.

2. Close in this view to the concept of things: once a thing is seen as the product of reification, it is seen as a product of reification which is not the 'same' thing at all (cf. Mirowski 1990).

3. One camp of anthropologists would, in any case, insist that however interested they are in cultural variation, anthropologists themselves cannot get away from the fact that what they select to call kinship always has some reference to biological fact. Gellner (1987) is eloquent on this.

4. Consanguines are joined by substance and affines are joined through marriage, traditionally the precondition for future substantial connections.

5. Thus one can refer to the decision 'to have a child' as a 'reproductive decision' (Birke *et al.* 1990 p. 13).

6. See Acknowledgements.

7. The whole issue of minority access to reproductive medicine from those with unconventional views on sexuality or family life has barely begun to address its potential ethnic dimensions in this country. For a class-sensitive account, see Seal (1990). It is also interesting in this context to read Birke *et al.* (1990 p. 251) who, in commenting on the Feversham Committee set up in 1960 to consider DI (then AID, and not yet part of the New Reproductive Technology syndrome), observe that it is Conservative thought that has particularly tended to assume that the social relations it favours are based on nature rather than social arrangement. The Committee viewed legitimacy as a 'legal recognition of a biological relationship'; a relationship with no biological basis could not be legitimated. One might observe in turn that 'social constructionist' arguments belong to the socialist enlightenment.

8. Dolgin (1990b p. 527) observes *apropos* the law applied to surrogacy disputes in

the United States that commissioning parents may appeal to the naturalness of their hope 'to replicate traditional family forms: to create nuclear families indistinguishable (except in origin) from old-fashioned American families'. (For my argument 'except in origin' could read 'except in kinship'.)

9. Stacey (1990) has commented on the biologisation of the family that is therefore reinforced. Contrast the traditional case of adoption in the past, where the closeness between parent and child is constituted on non-procreative criteria. When a commissioning couple seeks a substitution for some part of the procreative process itself, they preserve the symbolism of procreative closeness without enacting it.

10. Haimes (1990) argues that the controversy over anonymity in gamete donation can only be understood in relation to expectations about normative family structures.

11. It is a characteristic *of the kinship system*, I would argue, that built into the way people sustain relationships with one another is the supposition that much will turn on their preferences *vis-à-vis* specific persons. The classic studies of Firth, Hubert and Forge (1969) in England, and Rosser and Harris in Wales (1965) make this very evident. Some of the opprobrium which the nuclear family also draws as a 'trap' and constraint on people's lives (see Barrett and McIntosh 1982) is the other side of the value put on choice and preference.

12. Lifestyle may be an object of reproduction, a widespread factor in English versions of Euro-American kinship and with class overtones (e.g. Edwards 1991).

13. The desire to 'have' a child may be expressed by one person in the desire to pass on genetic identity, in another in the desire to bear and give birth (see Snowden and Mitchell 1981 p. pp. 40f). Where a couple is involved such expressions may also be transmuted into the desire to fulfil the desires of the partner. In Euro-American thought, the fulfilling of needs in this way is regarded as an important attribute of human nature (e.g. Quinn 1987 p. 189).

14. 'Always the case' in non-procreative and/or reproductive sexual relations. But that was taken care of in the distinction between sex and reproduction and/or procreation. The new distinction between reproduction and procreation will have different repercussions.

15. I am most grateful to Robert Snowden for directing me to these materials. The Report was an advisory document produced to assist the deliberations of the HFE Authority draft the counselling sections of its Code of Practice.

16. I do not comment on the manner in which scientific knowledge is transformed in its popular promulgation. The representation of embryo development in such a way as to make embryo research debatable in Parliament during the passage of the HFE Act offers one example.

17. One cultural parallel to this idea has already been given. Relations with them activated or not, persons involved in one's procreation are kin.

18. However inapposite the metaphor of 'programme', it has widespread popularity. The following is from the *Telegraph Magazine* (24 August 1991) report on the progress of the Human Genome Project: 'James Watson hopes that the entire genome will be decoded by the year 2006. By that time, it is expected that doctors will be able to provide any human being with a genetic "print-out". In other words, once all defective genes are decoded, it will in theory be possible to pinpoint the risks of hereditary disease faced by any individual . . . Geneticists

all agree that environment plays as large a part in the make-up of an individual as DNA. But will employers take the risk?'

19. See note 1. The basis of Lord Teviot's dismay with respect to the 'legal fiction' is this one can therefore continue to say that the importance of genealogy in medical research, especially research into the inheritance of genetic defects, grows every year as more and more illnesses, from colour blindness to fatal conditions, are found to be of an inherited nature. In relation to the comment that follows, I add that it is not that genealogical records will cease to matter ('Thus we can have a young, perfectly asymptomatic, individual who knows, from family history, that he has 50 per cent chance of having the normal gene') but that their centrality is displaced ('A genetic diagnosis could tell him whether he does possess the gene or not', Brenner 1990 p. 37).

20. The contrast between the influence of others and the autonomy of the individual is endemic to twentieth century Euro-American culture. Two American examples are given by (1) Dolgin (1990a,b) who draws the distinction between 'status' and 'contract' in pointing to contrasting and often competing sources of legal authority with respect to the family; (2) Ginsburg's (1989) account of the abortion debate in an American community which elicits the same contrast worked out through competing definitions of gender roles.

21. The relationship may even become contingent: when parents fail to provision adequately, the state may take over.

22. I am grateful to Jeanette Edwards for ethnographic evidence from another context to support this assertion. A theoretical case is made in Strathern (1992).

23. The two scenarios were articulated in another form in interviews conducted by Eric Hirsch; I am additionally grateful for Sarah Franklin's and Frances Price's insights here (see Acknowledgement).

24. Euro-Americans have various theories about the importance of the environment on the development of the individual organism, including about persons who are part of that environment. In that sense, other persons show their imprint on bodily constitution (and thus surrogacy contracts in the United States may include stipulations about the carrying mother's health routines). But the point is that the body *also* exists as an autonomous register of its own physiological processes, and we do not (culturally speaking) find it awkward to think of its system as internally programmed.

25. On the corresponding 'need for a child', see Franklin (1990). (Morgan and Lee (1991) go on to cite a counter argument that virtually suggests that if we get rid of socially induced needs we should be getting rid of society itself.)

ACKNOWLEDGEMENTS

This chapter was initially written during the lifetime of the ESRC – funded project ROOO 23 2537; the support of the ESRC is gratefully acknowledged, as is the expertise of other members of the project: Jeanette Edwards, Sarah Franklin, Eric Hirsch and Frances Price (see Edwards *et al.* 1993). I have appreciated David Schneider's comments on the first draft, as I do Sarah Franklin's.

REFERENCES

Barrett, M. and McIntosh, M. (1982), *The Anti-Social Family*, Verso, London

Birke, L., Himmelweit, S. and Vines, G. (1990), *Tomorrow's Child: Reproductive Technologies in the 90s*, Virago Press, London

Bloch, M. (1987), 'Descent and sources of contradiction in the representation of women and kinship'. In J. Collier and S. Yanagisako (eds.), *Gender and Kinship*, Stanford University Press

Brenner, S. (1991), 'Old ethics for new issues', *Science and Public Affairs* (The Royal Society, BAAS), August 1991

Davidoff, L. and Hall, C. (1987), *Family Fortunes: Men and Women of the English Middle Class 1780–1850*, Hutchinson, London

Dolgin, J. L. (1990a), 'Status and contract in feminist legal theory of the family: a reply to Bartlett', *Women's Rights Law Reporter*, XII, pp. 103–13

——'Status and contract in surrogate motherhood: an illumination of the surrogacy debate', *Buffalo Law Review*, XXXVIII, pp. 515–50

Edwards, J. (1991), 'Town houses or family homes?' Report to research group, La diversité culturelle des familles d'europe, Paris. Convenor, Martine Segalen

Edwards, J. *et al.* (1993), *Kinship in the Age of Assisted Conception*, Manchester University Press

Finch, J. (1989), *Family Obligations and Social Change*, Polity Press with Basil Blackwell, Cambridge

Firth, R., Hubert, J. and Forge, A. (1969), *Families and Their Relatives: Kinship in a Middle Class Sector of London*, Routledge & Kegan Paul, London

Franklin, S. (1990) 'Deconstructing "desperateness": the social construction of infertility in popular representations of new reproductive technologies', in M. McNeil *et al* (eds)., *The New Reproductive Technologies*, Macmillan, London

Gellner, F. (1987), *The Concept of Kinship and Other Essays*, Basil Blackwell, Oxford

Ginsburg, F. (1989), *Contested Lives: The Abortion Debate in an American Community*, University of California Press, Berkeley

Glover, J. *et al* (1989), *Fertility and the Family: The Glover Report on Reproductive Technologies to the European Commission*, Fourth Estate, London

Grobstein, C. (1990), 'Genetic manipulation and experimentation'. In D. R. Bromham, M. E. Dalton and J. C. Jackson (eds.), *Philosophical Ethics in Reproductive Medicine*, Manchester University Press

Haimes, E. (1990), 'Recreating the family? Policy considerations relating to the "new" reproductive technologies', in M. McNeil *et al.* (eds.), *The New Reproductive Technologies*, Macmillan, London

King's Fund Centre (1991), *Counselling for Regulated Infertility Treatments*, Reports of the King's Fund Centre Counselling Committee, London

Lamb, D. (1990), *Organ Transplants and Ethics*, Routledge, London

Mirowski, P. (1990), 'The rhetoric of modern economics', *History of the Human Sciences*, III, pp. 243–57

Morgan, D. and Lee, R. G. (1991), *Human Fertilisation and Embryology Act 1990: Abortion and Embryo Research, the New Law*, Blackstone Press Ltd, London

Price, F. V. (1990), 'The management of uncertainty in obstetric practice: ultrasonography, *in vitro* fertilisation and embryo transfer', in M. McNeil *et al.* (eds.), *The New Reproductive Technologies*, Macmillan, London

Quinn, N. (1987), 'Convergent evidence for a cultural model of American marriage', in N. Quinn and D. Holland (eds.), *Cultural Models in Language and Thought*, Cambridge University Press

Rabinow, P. (1990), 'Calton's regret'. Paper presented to the AAA Meetings, New Orleans, 1990 (manuscript)

Rapp, R. (1989), 'Chromosomes and communication: the discourse of genetic counselling', in I. M. Whiteford and M. L. Poland (eds.), *New Approaches to Human Reproduction: Social and Ethical Dimension*, Westview Press, Boulder

Rosser, C. and Harris, C. (1965), *The Family and Social Change: A Study of Family and Kinship in a South Wales Town*, Routledge & Kegan Paul, London

Schneider, D. M. (1968), *American Kinship: A Cultural Account*, Prentice Hall, Englewood Cliffs

——(1984), *A Critique of the Study of Kinship*, University of Michigan Press, Ann Arbor

Seal, V. (1990) *Whose Choice? Working Class Women and the Control of Fertility*, Fortress Books, London

Snowden, R. (1990), 'The family and artificial reproduction'. In D. R. Bromham, M. E. Dalton and J. C. Jackson (eds.), *Philosophical Ethics in Reproductive Medicine*, Manchester University Press

Snowden, R. and Mitchell, G. D. (1981), *The Artificial Family: A Consideration of Artificial Insemination by Donor*, Unwin, London

Stacey, M. (1990), 'Social dimensions of assisted reproduction'. Text of President's Day address, Sociology section, BAAS, Swansea

Strathern, M. (1992), *After Nature: English Kinship in the Late Twentieth Century*, Cambridge University Press

Warnock, M. (1985), *A Question of Life: The Warnock Report on Human Fertilisation and Embryology*, Basil Blackwell, Oxford

Wilson, P. ad Pahl, R. (1988), 'The changing sociological construct of the family', *Sociological Review*, pp. 233–66

PART TWO

Social and ethical issues in managing the use of high technology medicine

6

Ethical and economic aspects of life-saving and life-sustaining technologies

BRYAN JENNETT

Much of the burgeoning interest in the ethics and economics of health care can be ascribed to the increasing use of technology in medicine (Jennett 1986). Technology in general can be defined as the use of tools to assist in the tasks of diagnosis or of therapy. Many of these tools are of an increasingly sophisticated, high technology kind. Diagnostic technologies include imaging techniques (for example X-rays, Computerised Tomography (CT) Scans; Magnetic Resonance Imaging (MRI) Scans); endoscopes for direct inspect of internal organs; electronic monitoring of the heart, lungs, brain and nerves, and of blood flow in various organs; and examining the chromosomes to detect inherited abnormalities. Another currently widely used technology is the use of computers for processing information about individual patients, and to allow comparison with data on previous patients with similar conditions. In place of doctors' opinions about what is likely to happen, statistical probabilities can now often be provided for diagnosis and prognosis. Therapeutic technologies are mainly concerned with removing diseased parts – in this respect surgery is the oldest technology – or with substituting for lost function. Recent functional technologies include ventilators; kidney machines; heart pacemakers; and fertility techniques; as well as aids for disabled people.

Diagnosis can often be reached in less stressful and more accurate ways using technology, while therapeutic technologies can often save and extend lives of good quality, and improve the quality of life when death is not a threat. It might therefore be expected that the development of technological assistance would be a welcome development in medicine. However, these benefits have to be balanced against a variety of burdens. Because almost all technology needs teams of doctors in different disciplines, aided by specialised nurses, physicists and technicians, the patient is no longer alone with his or her doctor on the medical stage. Technology can therefore seem to distance doctors from their patients, replacing or reducing the touching and talking that used to be at the centre of the doctor-patient encounter. In this respect technology is sometimes suspected of having a dehumanising effect on medical practice. Doctors are also sometimes accused of being wedded to technology for its own sake, rather than employing it for the patient's benefit, particularly when the result is to prolong life of questionable quality.

ETHICAL ASPECTS OF THE USE OF MEDICAL TECHNOLOGIES

Issues about each of the four accepted principles of medical ethics frequently arise when technologies are used. The balance between *beneficence* and *non-maleficence* has always to be considered, as should the issue of *patient autonomy*. In relation to this latter principle the question has to be posed – has the patient had an opportunity to give informed consent to the initiation and continued use of each technology? Traditionally it is only surgery for which a signature by, or on behalf of, the patient has to be obtained, no matter how minor the procedure. Yet other life-saving and life-sustaining technologies can be of much more significance – for example those relating to resuscitation, ventilation, dialysis, or tube feeding. Most technologies are costly in terms of capital investment, consumables and specialised staff, making them limited in availability, as well as always competing with non-technological activities in health care. Thus it is important to consider the fourth ethical principle – *justice* – in the deployment of scarce resources. The question of justice often concerns technologies, both at the level of the provision of facilities or resources (macro-allocation), and of the selection of individual patients to be given the opportunity to benefit from them (micro-allocation).

ATTITUDES TO THE USE OF TECHNOLOGY

The variety and complexity of medical technologies is such that no-one can be fully informed about them all. That does not prevent strong views being held about their use which inevitably reflect the perspective of a particular observer. The debate may either be about the level of *provision* by health authorities of devices and staff, or about the *use* made of this provision by doctors (Jennett 1988c). Provision depends on reaching a balance between the claims of product champions for a given technology, and the perceptions of providers or purchasers of health care. Product champions are usually clinicians acting as advocates for particular patient groups. With newly emerging technologies, however, some clinicians may themselves have been involved in some aspect of an innovation, sometimes in collaboration with commercial interests. Where health care budgets are fixed, as in Britain, product champions and health authorities often appear to represent opposing vested interests – the one promoting and other tending to resist increased provision (Jennett 1989). Where market forces influence health care provision, however, hospital managers may wish to acquire a certain technology in order to attract patients from competing providers, as commonly occurs in the United States (see Chapter 7).

The main factor influencing the use of technologies has hitherto been the aggregated decisions of clinicians who treat individual patients. Where increased attention is being paid to the autonomy of patients, decisions made by them in their role as the ultimate consumers is becoming more important. Neither doctors nor patients can, however, make rational decisions unless there are good data about the efficacy and effectiveness of a technology in the specific circumstances in which it is applied. In practice such data about technology assessment are often lacking, so that decisions are often unduly influenced by the beliefs or prejudices of clinicians and patients. The extent of professional uncertainty about the value of many technologies is revealed by the wide variations observed in their rate of use, particularly by different surgeons and clinicians concerned with intensive care (Jennett 1992).

Apart from the role of those actively involved in the provision and use of medical technologies, other less immediately involved observers of such technologies often voice opinions about their use. The general public, made up entirely of patients (past, present or future), appears from surveys and other research to be ambivalent about the nature and role of medical technology. Some call for greater provision and more frequent use of certain technologies, perhaps based on unrealistic expectations of benefit from them. Others seem increasingly aware that certain technologies also have the capacity to harm, whilst some offer only limited benefits.

Public supporters of a particular medical technology are often associated with patient advocate groups for certain diseases, or those organisations associated with, and fund raising for, hospitals. Such groups and organisations may raise money for the purchase of equipment which they consider to be under-provided – and may be encouraged in this activity by relevant groups of clinicians. This process can operate almost independently of the circumstances necessary to ensure the effective operation of the technologies. Thus such fund raising may result in the acquisition of equipment (such as complex radiological installations or kidney dialysis machines) by hospitals which do not have enough patients to justify such technologies, or to enable personnel to develop and maintain adequate skills in their use. Additional pressures for the provision of high technology equipment may also come from politicians anxious to attract additional resources for their local hospital, or who feel compelled to support patient groups by which they have been lobbied.

The media have an important role in informing the public about medical technologies, and the increase in public awareness of the advantages and disadvantages of different technologies enhances the power of patients who wish to question the need for various procedures to which they are asked to consent. A moderating influence on the increasing use of high technology techniques comes from doctors in low technology specialties, who commonly hold that too great a proportion of health budgets goes to their colleagues using such resources. In drawing attention to the apparent inequity of allocations between different specialties, those clinicians in low technology specialties highlight the often limited value of some advanced high technologies. Psychiatrists, geriatricians, and others concerned with the care of chronic disabilities, are frequently supported in this view by those in public health medicine, who are concerned to achieve a more equitable balance of resource allocation between the acute and chronic sectors of health care. These 'doubting doctors' often seem unaware of the capacity that some technologies have for improving the quality of life of chronically disabled people and for reducing their dependency on others and, further, of the extent to which elderly people can benefit from many technologies. Implicit in the criticisms of these doctors is the belief that technological medicine is always unduly expensive, compared to other more efficient means of providing general health care.

THE ECONOMICS OF GENERAL SURGERY

Economics can be argued to be about balancing costs and benefits of alternative strategies (Jennett 1987). In health care it is usually easier to measure costs than benefits, and costs to the health service are more readily estimated than those borne by the patient and his or her family. Clinicians are usually inclined to accept more readily the study of cost-effectiveness of a technique or procedure than its cost-benefit analysis. *Cost-effectiveness* can be defined as the least costly means of achieving a specified beneficial end, whether diagnostic or therapeutic. Common measures of efficiency in surgery are, for example, the time waiting for a consultation; the interval until admission, and the time spent in hospital before and after surgery. Other measures which can be employed are the numbers of patients seen in each clinic, those operated on each week, or those admitted each year. Such performance indicators, however, deal only with the numbers of patients at each assessment point, and give no indication of whether the activities performed were appropriate – that is, those that were both necessary and effective.

On the other hand *cost-benefit analysis* concerns the allocative efficiency of resources, and in particular whether they would be better used in trying to achieve one end rather than another. Because such analysis involves choosing ends rather than means, it inevitably questions whether the balance of work in a specialist unit, or a hospital or health authority is appropriate. Would it be better, for example, if surgeons spent less time treating advanced life-threatening conditions and were therefore able to deal with more patients with conditions that do not threaten life, but where surgery could greatly improve the quality of life of such patients (Jennett 1991)? It is probable that many surgeons who have long waiting lists for elective operations, such as hernia repair, may expend an undue amount of their resources on operations for patients with hopeless conditions. Many of these latter patients may be admitted as emergencies, and may also be elderly with advanced cancer. There are also serious questions about the balance between cardiac bypass surgery, renal dialysis and genetic screening, given finite resources devoted to health care. Such an approach requires the monetary evaluation of benefits. However, few of these benefits may involve readily ascertainable financial gains, such as patients' improved earning capacity.

To ascribe monetary values to apparently intangible benefits such as to the relief of pain, or to the resolution of anxiety and uncertainty, requires common and agreed judgements about how quality of life can be measured. Such agreement will be difficult to obtain. Nonetheless the attempt to undertake this assessment has the advantage of making clear how much weight is generally attached to value judgements about the quality of life, compared to more readily ascertainable monetary benefits and burdens.

The measure most commonly used in cost-benefit analysis is the number of years of good life that are gained as a result of a given intervention. The outcome of treatment is compared with that expected either with alternative methods of treatment, or with no treatment at all. The difference between the expected number of unacceptable or bad outcomes (death or disability) without treatment, and those occurring after treatment, is the product of the intervention. This benefit must be qualified by life expectancy, leading to the controversial concept of quality-adjusted life-years (QALYs) (Cubbon 1991). Interestingly most of the controversy about the construction and use of this measure has been in the context of medical ethics – as though ethics and economics were assumed to be in conflict (Harris 1987, 1991; Smith 1987). In fact the dictates of good ethics and good economics often coincide and indeed the QALY can be regarded as a tool that allows medical practice to take account of the fourth principle of medical ethics – maintaining justice or equity in the allocation and use of health care resources.

THE COSTS OF TECHNOLOGY: THE EXAMPLE OF SURGERY

The decisions of surgeons to operate result in the deployment of substantial revenue resources – for example the time of surgeons, and that of anaesthetists, nurses and technicians in operating theatres, and the use of beds and investigative facilities. Major surgery often entails a commitment to costly post-operative intensive care, while certain procedures use expensive items such as artificial joints, heart valves or vascular prostheses. Elective surgery is therefore very susceptible to limitations in the supply of consumables or of staff, largely because it is easy for purchasers and providers to estimate the financial implications of surgery. This issue makes surgical patients particularly vulnerable to the withdrawal or postponement of services whenever there is a need to contain short term costs. Occasionally hospital managements in Britain may declare in advance how many of a particular type of operation can be performed (that is, will be funded). More often overall resources are reduced, and the surgeons are left to assign priorities to different types of procedure and to choose between patients, within the available budget. With the move to provider/purchaser arrangements in the British National Health Service these decisions are likely to become more explicit and visible.

Most surgical costing is based on estimating the cost *per day* for a patient in a normal surgical bed, and for time spent by a patient in an intensive care bed (commonly about five times greater). Costs per hour in the operating theatre can also be calculated, with a higher rate for night or emergency use. By aggregating these costs it is possible to calculate an average cost per procedure. Even ascertaining average costs of this kind is complex and difficult. Yet another problem is the wide range of costs incurred by different patients with the same condition, according to severity of illness. Costs are usually much higher in the first few days after admission, because of investigations, surgery and post-operative intensive care. Thus the economic benefits of reducing length of hospital stay by sending patients home sooner can easily be exaggerated – if they are based on average costs per day.

Similarly focusing only on the costs incurred within the surgical unit during an episode of treatment ignores other medical costs before and after such an episode (Jennett and Pickard 1992). There may have been investigations performed on an out-patient basis or undertaken by another speciality (e.g. cardiology or neurology). Organ transplantation also involves substantial ongoing costs in drugs and surveillance, making it appropriate to quote 'first year costs' for survivors. Less complex surgery may appear to have been made less expensive for the hospital budget by means of early discharge or day surgery. However, nurses and doctors in the community are then involved in procedures normally undertaken in hospital such as removing stitches and giving post-operative support and advice, which needs to be taken into account, as well as other associated costs, such as specialist transport. Therefore the new arrangements for funding health care in the National Health Service run the risk of merely transferring costs from one budget to another rather than cutting them.

Patients with disabilities requiring remedial services also incur considerable post-hospital costs – whether this is provided at home or by attendance at a rehabilitation unit. When life-saving treatment results in prolonged survival with severe disability, much larger economic costs may be incurred over the subsequent years of dependence than would have resulted from cost-benefit calculations in relation to an early death. One example of such a situation is when resuscitation after acute brain damage from injury or cardiac arrest results in averting death but leads to survival with severe brain damage (Jennett 1990). Even when these long term costs are included it is all too easy to count the hospital costs only of those patients who were successfully diagnosed or treated by a given technology. However, expenditure incurred on the many patients who had negative investigations or unsuccessful treatment must enter the cost calculation as well as that for each patient counted as a success.

THE PATIENT AND THE FAMILY AND HIGH TECHNOLOGY MEDICINE

Lost earnings to the patient and their care-givers from their condition and its management, together with the added expense of travelling for treatment, or for visiting, are relatively easily calculated. But the personal burdens of treatment borne by the patient are even more important. With surgery there is the immediate risk of peri-operative mortality and of complications. The operation may also fail to cure or even to improve the condition. Moreover some surgical procedures have inevitable consequences for patients' quality of life even when surgery has been successful and uncomplicated. This may apply, for example, to the mutilation and dysfunction associated with mastectomy or the amputation of a limb. The surgeon has therefore a duty to present to the patient the benefits and burdens of the surgery proposed, and of alternative treatments. The surgeon may also discuss the relative merits of surgery now, compared with postponing it, and of different surgical procedures.

THE BENEFITS OF TREATMENT

It is not enough to claim as a benefit of technological treatment that the patient is likely to have a good outcome. It has also to be shown that this is a significantly better outcome than was predicted either without treatment or with an alternative treatment that might have been less costly or risky. Before deciding whether a particular intervention is 'worthwhile' there is thus a need to consider how many patients benefit, how much they benefit, and for how long they benefit (Williams 1985). There are therefore two crucial steps in deciding if a treatment is effective – the assessment of the actual outcome, and the prediction of what the outcome would have been without that treatment. There is much to be said for assessment of outcomes by a third person, or by the patient themselves, using structured interviews or questionnaires and scoring systems. Generic questionnaires, such as the Nottingham Health Profile, or the Scale of Wellbeing, can be used to supplement data that are specific to the treated condition. In this context it is important that the chosen outcomes should measure what patients want out of treatment, rather than reflect the technical aims of doctors alone.

THE INAPPROPRIATE USE OF TECHNOLOGIES

Most criticisms of a technology prove to be of its inappropriate use (Angell 1990), which is surprisingly common even where resources for technology are restricted. There are few technologies that are never of benefit, but even the best technology can only be of benefit to selected patients. Five types of inappropriate use of technology have been identified. Use may be *unnecessary* because the patient's condition is insufficiently serious to justify it. This may apply to many diagnostic procedures as well as to much of the monitoring in coronary and intensive care units and in obstetric delivery rooms. In addition the use of a technology may be *unsuccessful*, because the patient's condition is too far advanced to respond to that intervention. This applies particularly to rescue surgery for advanced cancer and to intensive care for terminally ill patients (Jennett and Buxton 1990). Less absolute types of inappropriate use may occur when the use of a technology is deemed to be *unkind*, because it prolongs life which is of poor quality; or when it is *unsafe*, because the expected complications outweigh the anticipated benefits of its use. Lastly the use of a technology may be deemed *unwise*, because it diverts resources from alternative health care activities that would bring more benefit to other patients. The first four of these inappropriate uses offend the ethical principle of disproportion between the probability of beneficence and that of non-maleficence. A sixth type of inappropriate use might be when it is *unwanted*, because it is against the patient's wishes, and thereby denies his or her autonomy.

There are several reasons why doctors so often manage to ignore the claims of both ethics and economics, even when these coincide (Williams 1992). The most important reason why they so often indulge in inappropriate use of technologies in hospital is lack of knowledge about the benefits and burdens of applying a given technology in particular circumstances – given the age of the patient and the severity of his or her condition (Jennett 1988b). This is often blandly described as professional uncertainty, but this could be more bluntly termed ignorance. There may be no data available about what to expect from the intervention; or that data may not be known to the decision-maker at the time. Sometimes the doctor may choose to ignore available data, either because he does not think they apply in this particular case, or because intellectually or intuitively he disbelieves them.

However, clinicians confronted with patients who are critically ill, or who have distressing symptoms or a dreaded diagnosis, have a natural wish to respond positively. This may account for the decision to employ technologies inappropriately, especially in emergency situations, perhaps influenced by the perceived or supposed expectations of the patient and the family, and of other doctors and nurses. Examples are cardiopulmonary resuscitation when cardiac arrest occurs in a patient already hopelessly ill, or surgical intervention for someone with advanced and incurable cancer (Jennett 1990). Whatever the reasons, decision-making in acute hospitals is carried out in the presence of a host of witnesses. It is easy to state the general principles that it is bad medicine to persist with futile treatment, and that no patient has a right to futile treatment. Examples are continuing with artificial feeding of a patient with irrecoverable brain damage who can never regain consciousness, or with ventilation in a patient with irrecoverable organ failure. But some doctors are reluctant to limit treatment when confronted with a seriously ill patient. As an excuse for their inappropriate actions they may claim uncertainty about the prognosis, or the possibility that a technological intervention might help, even when all the evidence is against both these assertions. This behaviour is not peculiar to the affluent West. In Eastern Europe I have seen an intensive care unit entirely filled with cases with a hopeless prognosis, whilst in the ward there were many patients with curable conditions, often two to a bed, receiving minimal care. And a student of mine reported in Papua New Guinea that he observed people who would insist on surgical intervention for a terminally ill relative even when told that the prognosis was very poor, and the surgical intervention would be completely ineffective.

In reviewing the reasons (or excuses) for over-treatment of patients by technologies it would be disingenuous not to include the fear, whether real or apparent, of subsequent legal proceedings. In the United States so-called defensive medicine may be inevitable but there is not a valid basis for such practice in Europe. A useful defence against such concern is the development of guidelines or consensus statements that indicate the general circumstances in which decisions may properly be made to limit treatment (Stanley 1989). These would include a medical decision that treatment was futile, a combined decision by doctor and patient (or family) that treatment was disproportionately burdensome in regard to expected benefit, or that the patient had requested no treatment – either personally or by the mechanism of an advanced directive.

TOWARDS THE MORE APPROPRIATE USE OF TECHNOLOGIES

More rational and effective use of technologies is likely to develop only when more data are available about their effects, and it becomes accepted ethical practice for doctors to take due account of such data when making decisions. A strategy of technology assessment needs first to identify effective technologies, and then to determine the limits of appropriate use. Before considering the affordable level of provision of effective technologies, some form of economic appraisal is also required. Pressures from two sources are likely to lead to an increased demand for technology assessment. One is from patients who need this information in order to be able to express preferences and participate in decisions; and to be protected from ineffective, unacceptable and futile technologies. The other is from providers who wish to fund only effective established technologies when appropriately used, and to support the introduction of new technologies only when assured that they will be systematically assessed during their initial period of use.

Strict trials are the rule for drugs, not only because licensing depends on adequate trials having been carried out, but because the considerable expense that assessment entails is commonly met by the pharmaceutical industry. By contrast there is no restriction on the introduction of surgical innovations or of new techniques in intensive care. Even for new devices, like CT and MRI, there is no requirement to test beyond safety. Randomised trials are the ideal method of assessment for drugs, but ethical, economic and practical considerations limit their use for some of the technologies used to rescue severely ill patients. The next best approach to more appropriate application of technologies is to maintain an accurate prospective audit of the use of such technologies, and of the outcomes when used for different types of patient. It is easier to determine the short term value of interventions that aim at averting an immediate threat to life, or to relieve symptoms, than to evaluate their effect on the patient's life as a whole. Thus an intensive care unit may claim a mortality within the unit of only 20% of admissions, but another 20% may die before leaving hospital and another 20% during the year after leaving hospital. Assessment of effectiveness therefore requires adequate definition of the objectives of therapeutic intervention within an appropriate time frame.

Decision-making is often difficult in rescue medicine (emergency surgery, unplanned intensive care and resuscitation). Such patients fall into three groups. Some have suffered sudden illness or accident and for them all must be done initially in the way of life-saving and life-sustaining measures, unless (or until) it is certain that the situation is hopeless. It may be some time before relatives can be consulted about the patient's previous medical history and his attitude to rescue procedures. The second group are those undergoing planned surgery or other procedures in hospital who have developed a serious complication. Much is already known about these patients, and the possibility of such a crisis may already have been discussed with them. Lastly there are patients with chronic, progressive conditions who suffer a predictable crisis or relapse. The probability of such an eventuality should have been discussed with the patient and the family, and the possibility raised that it may be better not to intervene with rescue measures. These situations are made easier if patients have made an advance directive, such as a living will. With foresight much unjustified technological intervention could be avoided or at least limited – resulting in more compassionate and more economic care.

In practice the doctor who has to decide what to do in a crisis may know little about the patient's previous medical history, and nothing about his attitude to rescue. Inevitably there is a tendency to inappropriate over-treatment, which may begin a cycle of commitment that is difficult to break. Many doctors and nurses find it more difficult to withdraw treatment that has been started than to withhold it in the first place. Yet in some patients it is only after a trial period of resuscitation or intensive care that it becomes clear that there will be no immediate or lasting benefit. However, it is one thing to refer a patient with advanced cancer to a hospice a few weeks or months before death, but more difficult to deal appropriately with a terminal crisis resulting in emergency admission to an acute hospital in the middle of the night.

Intensive care units offer a range of technological rescue options, both to save and to sustain life. These include ventilators, drugs to maintain blood pressure and cardiac action, transfusion of blood, artificial provision of fluids and nutrition, and haemodialysis. There are also many monitoring techniques used to identity the technical needs of a patient and his response to treatment, none of which is free of risk, so that they may sometimes do more harm than good. Moreover the continued activity around the patient, the lights on all night, the witnessing or overhearing of crises affecting nearby patients, all contrive to make an intensive care unit a disturbing environment for a conscious patient, as well as for his or her relatives. Unless there is definite benefit from being there, it is no place to be.

The numbers and high level of training of nurses in intensive care units makes the daily costs about five times greater than in an ordinary ward. Both humanity and economics may therefore dictate that a decision to withdraw intensive care be made as soon as possible. To do so only after a week or more of expensive futile treatment is hardly a decision at all. The failure to decide to withdraw treatment from a hopeless patient is in effect a decision to deny treatment to a less severely affected patient who could benefit, given that intensive care is a scarce resource (which it almost everywhere is, in availability of staff, if not of finance.)

GUIDELINES FOR THE MORE APPROPRIATE USE OF TECHNOLOGY

My theme has been the frequency with which technologies that can be of undoubted benefit in some circumstances are used inappropriately. This offends one or more of the principles of medical ethics, including a waste of scare resources. Improvement might come from the availability of better data from the assessment of technology, but decision-makers could still ignore such assessments if they felt a conflict with some vague concept of good medical practice, associated with the principle of sanctity of life. There may also be a reluctance to choose between patients on the basis of the relative benefits that treatment might confer on each, preferring to leave 'the choice' to be based on 'first come first served', which is in effect a lottery. Other clinicians accept the need for systematic selection, but in practice do so by implicit criteria which are seldom openly discussed.

Whether decisions are being made about elective surgery or dialysis, or admission to, or discharge from intensive care, there is considerable virtue in having written guidelines which make selection policies more explicit. If the principles of selection have been stated by a national professional society, or a consensus conference, medical staff will be reassured that local policies are in accord with good practice in the medical and nursing professions. It is, however, essential that guidelines are compatible with local circumstances and are agreed by local staff. Developed in this way guidelines have the advantage of resulting from discussion outside the emotional context of any individual case, and of representing a group judgement on appropriate criteria. Quite apart from the detailed guidance they may provide, they indicate that decisions about the use of technology should depend more on stated policies, than on personal intuition or the prejudices of individual clinicians.

Openly declaring policies makes it possible to debate and change them if necessary. Common fears that the operation of guidelines will be associated with insufficient account being taken of the needs of individual patients must be balanced by the reality that without such guidelines wide variations in practice will occur, thus offending against one or more of the principles of medical ethics.

CONCLUSION

Technologies have great potential for reducing avoidable death and disability; for improving the quality of life, and for prolonging lives of good quality. To fulfil that potential requires more knowledge about the effects of technology, and a great willingness to reach agreement about optimal practice given the present state of knowledge – however incomplete that knowledge may be. This approach holds out the best hope for a more rational, more humane, and more economic use of medical technologies, in accordance with the ethical principles indicated at the outset of this discussion.

REFERENCES

Angell, M. (1990), 'Prisoners of technology: the case of Nancy Cruzan', *New England Journal of Medicine*, CCCXXII, pp. 1226–8

Cubbon, J. (1991), 'The principle of QALY maximisation as the basis for allocating health care resources;, *Journal of Medical Ethics*, XVII, pp. 181–4

Harris, J. (1987), 'QALYfying the value of life', *Journal of Medical Ethics*, XIII, pp. 117–23

—— 'Unprincipled QALYs: a response to Cubbon', *Journal of Medical Ethics xvii*, p. 185–8

Jennett, B. (1986), *High Technology Medicine: Benefits and Burdens*, Oxford University Press

—— 'Are ethics and economics incompatible in health care?', *Proceedings of the Royal College of Physicians of Edinburgh*, XVII, pp. 190–5

—— (1988a) 'Balancing benefits and burdens of surgery', *British Medical Bulletin,* XLIV, pp. 499–513

—— (1988b) 'HTM and the elderly', in M. Wells and C. Freer (eds.), *Health Problems of an Ageing Population,* Macmillan, London, pp. 177–90

—— (1988c), 'Assessment of clinical technologies: importance for provision and use', *International Journal of Technology Assessment in Health Care,* IV, pp. 435–45

—— (1989), 'Quality of care and cost containment in the US and UK', *Theoretical Medicine,* X, pp. 207–15

—— (1990), 'Is intensive care worthwhile?', *Care of the Critically Ill* III, pp. 85–8

—— (1991) 'Decisions to limit the use of technologies that save or sustain life', *Proceedings of the Royal College of Physicians of Edinburgh,* XX, pp. 407–15

—— (1992), 'Health technology assessment', *British Medical Journal,* CCCV, pp. 67–8

Jennett, B. and Buxton, M. (1990), 'When is treatment for cancer economically justified?', *Journal of the Royal Society of Medicine,* LXXXIII, pp. 25–8

Jennett, B. and Pickard, J. (1992), 'Economic aspects of neurosurgery', in *Advances and Technical Standards in Neurosurgery,* XIX, pp. 123–43

Smith, A. (1987), 'Qualms about QALYs', *Lancet* II, pp. 1134–6

Stanley, J. M. (1989) 'The Appleton Consensus: suggested international guidelines for decisions to forgo life-prolonging medical treatment', *Journal of Medical Ethics,* XV, pp. 129–36

Williams, A. (1985), 'Economics of coronary bypass grafting', *British Medical Journal,* CCXCI, pp. 326–9

—— (1992), 'Cost effective analysis: is it ethical?', *Journal of Medical Ethics* XVII pp. 7–11

7

The social consequences of the development of the artificial heart

THOMAS PRESTON

In the absence of an implantable artificial brain, the fully implantable artificial heart would seem to be the ultimate in medical technology. The story of the permanent artificial heart, as it unfolded in the United States in the 1980s, is a story of the technological imperative, of individual and institutional gain, and of corporate power and profit. It is a story of high technology escaped from the bounds of public accountability, and serves as a warning of the potential abuse of medical technology.

In the artificial heart programme in the United States, sponsored primarily by the National Institutes of Health (NIH), only once was there a serious assessment of related nontechnical, or societal issues. The NIH have sponsored four or five assessment panels over the 25 years and more that they have supported research on the artificial heart, but only one, convened in 1972, went beyond the circumscribed bounds of technology analysis (National Heart, Lung and Blood Institute 1973 pp. 14–16).

The NIH had intended to restrict the panel to recommendations for the use of a device reliable enough to function free of problems for 10 years, but the panel took an expanded view of its charge. It called attention to the public's asserted right to 'reject any particular technological development on the ground that, even though it may benefit some members of society, it is inconsistent with values that society as a whole considers paramount' (National Heart, Lung and Blood Institute 1973 p. 2). It is not mere coincidence that this was the only panel not composed entirely of, or not dominated by, engineers and medical researchers.

THE ARTIFICIAL HEART AND QUALITY OF LIFE ISSUES

The 1972 NIH panel acknowledged that technology frequently has been misused for the purposes of prolonging life without regard for quality, and prophetically asked what would happen if the artificial heart fell below expectations and left patients alive but gravely impaired. Panel members raised the spectre of patients maintained in states just short of death, and forecast that doctors might be reluctant to deny patients extended life at the cost of decreased quality. They questioned the technological imperative and pointed out the difficulty in turning back from a technological *fait accompli.*

The 1972 NIH panel also pointed out potential disadvantages to society as a whole, regardless of short term benefit to individuals. Unrehabilitated patients might become a burden to their families and to the community as well. As the panel report poignantly put it: 'Perhaps the worst possible outcome would be for the device to work just well enough to induce patients to want it – so that they could see their grandchildren grow up, for example – but not well enough to prevent the typical recipient from substantially burdening others' (National Heart, Lung and Blood Institute 1973 pp. 71–2).

In thinking about whether we want the artificial heart we must consider first its technologic capabilities, and what kind of life it will provide. Kidney dialysis is intermittent, and failure of the haemodialysis machine necessitates only a move to another machine, but the artificial heart must be perfect to the point of never failing without sufficient warning time. The artificial pacemaker provides a good analogy for this point. Over the first twenty years of development there were repeated failures due to a number of causes, most of which were not anticipated by medical and engineering investigators. Pacemakers are an order of magnitude simpler than artificial hearts, having only one moving part and requiring one millionth the power to run, yet during the first five years of pacemaker implantations the average time before clinical failure was six months, and many patients had ten or more operations to correct device failure. When a pacemaker stops suddenly, as they still do, the consequences are seldom serious and deaths are extremely rare, but the cessation of artificial heart function will be an emergency of the greatest magnitude.

The clinical experiences of the five permanent implant recipients of the Jarvik–7 artificial heart provide a most disturbing profile (Gil 1989 pp. 24–31). All five patients suffered severe infections within 30 days of receiving the device, a complication that may well persist even without connections through the skin to outside power sources. All patients suffered strokes, and all but one, who died suddenly of a massive stroke, suffered severe physical and mental incapacitations. Indeed, the clinical failure of the artificial heart programme resulted not from an adverse technological assessment, or from concerns of the surgeons undertaking the implants, but from a public perception of the terrible quality of life of recipients of the device.

Moreover, if future models function longer, they will only defer the time of failure. Sudden failure of an artificial heart could result in death or irreversible brain damage within 10 to 15 seconds. If and when the point is reached that artificial heart patients leave the protective environment of a hospital, disasters will be encountered due to unanticipated failures at times and places where patients cannot receive immediate emergency treatment. It will take a decade or more after the start of routine implantations for investigators to learn what such problems are and how to deal with them. However, artificial hearts will always run the risk of sudden failure. Thus serious thought must be given as to whether this kind of existence should be promoted.

THE COST OF THE ARTIFICIAL HEART

The potential cost of the artificial heart, in dollars for the use of medical resources, is very substantial and could be described as staggering. For heart transplantation, practised for two decades, the average cost in the United States now exceeds $100,000, with annual follow-up costs of about $12,000. The artificial heart has an additional financial cost: the development of the equipment. Since 1964, federal contracts and grants for development of artificial hearts have reached in total about $300 million, with more funds being allocated through private sources (Preston 1988 pp. 91–126).

The heart and related equipment that Barney Clark received on December 1, 1982, cost about $16,000, exclusive of development, and the manufacturers project a similar price, adjusted for inflation, even after mass production. Newer models may cost more. It is difficult to predict the average hospital and professional cost of future artificial heart implantation because the average duration of hospitalization and number and type of complications is not known. Clark's expenses were covered by research funds or donated by the hospital, but if his hospital bill and doctors' fees were calculated in the usual itemized manner, the price was approximately $250,000 (Preston 1988 p. 122).

With the air powered artificial heart that Clark received, and its potential for leaking air and causing infection, it would be unrealistic to calculate an average initial implantation cost of less than $100,000 per patient. However, many advocates of the artificial heart have equated the cost to that of common artery bypass surgery, or about $25,000–30,000 per patient. But this is overly optimistic. The Barney Clark case suggests that there are markedly increased costs for the artificial heart, due not only to the cost of the equipment, but especially due to the cost of prolonged intensive care, and for re-operations for repair of mechanical failures.

It is not possible to estimate what the cost of long term follow-up for Barney Clark would have been. However, one patient, Murray Haydon, lived more than a year, most of that time in an intensive care unit attached to a respirator. The hospital estimates that Barney Clark's family would have spent $2,700 to adapt an apartment to the patient's needs – this of course being in addition to the cost of moving from Seattle to Salt Lake City. In Clark's case anonymous donors offered accommodation, but if artificial hearts were to be implanted on a large scale, the public could not be expected to donate tens of thousands of apartments a year. Follow-up costs, beginning from the time the patient first leaves the hospital after receiving the implant, include medicines, doctors' checkups, laboratory tests, and costs for re-hospitalization for any problems secondary to the artificial heart.

In the light of all these possible costs, it is crucial to undertake a realistic estimate of the overall costs of the adoption of the policy of artificial heart implantation. However, calculation of the costs depends on yet another currently unknown variable – the number of patients who would receive the heart if it were to be developed to the point of reliability. Estimates vary from 20,000 to 200,000 such patients a year in the United States (Preston 1988 p. 99). At a cost of $250,000 per patient at 1993 costs (a conservative estimate for implantation and follow-up), the outlay comes to between $5 and $50 billion a year, exclusive of development costs.

The size of these costs raises several very important questions – for example, who will pay? Only a very wealthy individual could finance his/her own personal costs, and the major insurance companies are unlikely to fund such an expensive technology. The government would be left to pay. As public demand for new medical technologies is always unrealistically high, as the device becomes more reliable, more and more patients will clamour for it. It will be almost impossible to deny the demand for its widespread use. This was the case for haemodialysis, which the government now funds at a cost of several billion dollars a year. The combination of commercial enterprises wanting to sell the heart and physicians wanting to use it will dovetail with public demand. As was learnt from the experience of dialysis, the estimated costs of providing the universal application of a new technology are almost always far too low.

There are other important policy implications. Federal spending in one area effectively precludes spending in another: the budget is limited, meaning de facto rationing of competing government services. Within the budget of the Department of Health and Human Services, an expenditure of $1 billion a year on artificial hearts means one billion dollars that is not available for other services. If the Medicare and Social Security programmes must finance artificial hearts, the funds must be diverted from other services provided by those agencies. The only other alternative is that they will have to come from general funds, which means less resources for other non- medical programmes. At a time of serious limitation of Medicare benefits, large costs for artificial hearts would mean fewer, or no benefits for many patients. Even in the private sector, spending for artificial hearts would result either in unacceptable insurance premium increases or decreases of other services.

If the United States government embarks on a policy of spending billions on a technology which, if perfected, is predicted to prolong the life of the recipient by an average of 0.6 years – and by extrapolation extend the mean life expectancy of the American population by only a few days – it raises the serious ethical issue of resource allocation in society. For example, the evidence suggests that the allocation of far less resources could improve infant mortality to a level which raised mean life expectancy far more than that which could be achieved with the artificial heart, thereby casting grave doubts on the social justice of spending billions of dollars on artificial hearts for a relatively few patients. Even within the field of cardiovascular diseases there is little evidence to support the value of unrestrained expenditure on artificial hearts. Such expenditure would inevitably act to the detriment of other relevant programmes. Several studies have shown the potential benefit of community-wide programmes aimed at reducing so-called risk factors for heart disease – lowering cholesterol levels, instituting proper exercise, controlling blood pressure, and educating the public to stop smoking. The exact benefit of these programmes is not known, nor is their cost known on a nationwide basis, but for an equivalent cost they would probably be more effective in reducing disability from heart disease and in prolonging life than the implantation of artificial hearts. Similarly, funds spent on basic research into the cause of heart disease, such as the cardiomyopathy that affected Barney Clark, might well be more productive than spending resources on artificial hearts which in themselves do nothing to prevent or alleviate the disease requiring the treatment. Given a choice, many might favour spending scarce funds on social rather than medical programmes that improve quality of life.

THE TECHNOLOGICAL ASSESSMENT OF THE ARTIFICIAL HEART

Dr Robert Jarvik, in a *Scientific American* article, said, 'Neither the Jarvik–7 nor any of the several other total artificial hearts being developed is yet ready to permanently replace a human heart, even on a trial basis' (Jarvik 1981). Yet, less than two years later and with no substantive improvement of the technology, he and his team implanted such a heart as the first in what they intended to become an accepted national if not global medical policy.

Although it might be argued that the Utah team that undertook the first 'permanent' implant was motivated probably more by the potential of institutional, personal and financial gain as much as disinterested research, their initial public defence was along other lines. Foremost in their arguments was the technological imperative – 'that which can be done must be done'. Dr Chase Peterson of the University of Utah defended the first implantation not as a beneficial technology, or even as research, but as a 'legitimate idea,' and added, 'If this country somehow ever got the notion that an idea is dangerous, we would be in the intellectual Dark Ages' (Preston 1985).

The Utah team brushed aside questions about the future by saying, in effect, that we must first find out how well the artificial heart works, or we will never know its potential and thus may lose a life-saving technology. By implication the social and economic problems attending such a development could wait until later. William DeVries, the surgeon who operated on Barney Clark, answered questions about societal issues by saying, 'We have to find out if it works and then debate what it costs.' (Preston 1985 p. 7). But in a real sense, the Utah team chose to bypass assessment of its technology by proclaiming it as a successful and necessary *therapy* at the time of its first use. The assertion – that the Jarvik–7 model of the artificial heart was of therapeutic value – edged the advocates on to shakier ethical ground by making dubious claims of clinical success. Virtually the first state-ment Dr DeVries made after the first implant had been undertaken was that Barney Clark would have been dead within hours had he not received the artificial heart (Preston 1985 p. 5). Other physicians might well have argued that life actually was shortened by the use of the procedure. But by predicting Barney Clark's imminent demise, and saying that they had extended his life, the team precluded the most serious objection to the implantation of the artificial heart.

The team also made general claims of therapeutic benefit for the artificial heart. DeVries, in explaining his move from Salt Lake City to Louisville, said, 'I don't like to see people die while I wait for the red tape.' The claim locked the team into producing a patina of thera-peutic success (or a denial of any setbacks) covering each clinical development. This framework foreclosed the far more legitimate option of proceeding with the development of the artificial heart strictly as a research project, with the quiet approval of the medical community, and to relative indifference in the media. Instead, the team's primary goal was a substantiation of their claim: to be 'vindi-cated', as Dr DeVries put it (Preston 1985 p. 5). However, most would argue that good research needs no vindication.

A critical point here is informed consent by patients to the use of a highly experimental technology. Doctors can always 'sell' an oper-ation to a dying and desperate patient under the rubric of therapy, and if a team of medical investigators backed by venture capitalists and a publicity-seeking institution choose to disguise the true nature of experimentation, the patient and his/her family are deceived. In this regard, the only watchdog in relation to the initial implantations, the Institutional Review Board (IRB) first at Utah and later at Louisville, can be argued to have failed to protect its patients.

The process of implantation of an artificial heart into Barney Clark in particular illustrates several issues relevant to the introduction, and evaluation of such new medical technologies. Most importantly, the Barney Clark saga was as much an experiment in the use of the public media to market a medical technology, as it was a scientific experiment. No medical event had been so extensively and intensively covered as was this one, and never before was there so much debate over reports in the media and the purposes for which they were used. If medicine was coming of age in its use of public relations, the Barney Clark epic marked the beginning of the deliberate employment of reporting to influence public acceptance that a medical 'advance' had occurred.

Once Barney Clark had his operation on December 2, 1982, the story shifted from the humdrum reporting of animal testing to the drama of a human patient with the bionic heart. For months those involved in public relations at the University of Utah had prepared for what they had anticipated and created – a media blitz. Reporters (of which hundreds notified in advance came from all over the world) were each given a pack of background papers and articles describing the Utah heart and its process of development. Immediately after the operation, hospital spokesmen made regular announcements and were responsive and accommodating to the media interest. The surgical team was available for questioning. The reporters were persistent, and committed to the story (Preston 1988 p. 119).

For the most part the media reported the event as drama, not as medical experimentation. Understandably, the focus of the press and the Utah spokesmen was on the personal stories of the players in the drama. In the previous most notable medical media spectacular, swashbuckling surgeon Christiaan Barnard was the centre of attention. This time it appeared that the surgeon, DeVries, at the centre of the implantation of the artificial heart was too reticent to make good media copy. The media turned instead to the patient who had dared to sacrifice himself to the experiment. Barney Clark had media appeal, and instantly schoolchildren across America knew about him and his devoted wife, Una Loy Clark. The operation was likened to the landing on the moon, and Barney Clark, pioneer and explorer, was compared to Columbus. Although some reporters raised hard questions about the use of technology, its cost, the question of informed consent, and the rationing of scarce resources, the event in general was presented to the media and duly reported to the public as a remarkable technological breakthrough, with all the trappings of a live soap opera.

For the first few days after Barney Clark's implant, hospital spokesmen and the surgical team fed news to the assembled reporters. Spokesmen made statements such as 'He's doing better, if anything, than a standard (heart) bypass patient.' (Preston 1983). DeVries said Barney Clark could leave the hospital 'within a few weeks', and Jarvik said that tests of the artificial heart showed that it was capable of operating for at least four and a half years. Even Dr Willem Kolff, the true inventor of the heart and usually very cautious in commenting on its use, made wild predictions that artificial heart recipients would be barred from marathons within fifteen years because they would be too strong for other competitors (Bernstein 1984). These early statements, eagerly swallowed by a public hungry for good news, produced the first impressions of an uncertain, perilous experiment of a device that had sustained cloistered life for an average of two and a half months in animals.

About ten days after the first implant, it appeared that the clinical team soured on the media which had so willingly publicized the event, and began to perceive it as inimical to their interests. There was growing internal concern about releasing too much information, and a collective desire of the team emerged to reduce the degree of media interest in the story. Hospital spokesmen erroneously denied that Clark, a Mormon, was a long standing cigarette smoker. It became clear that his doctors had not fully appreciated the seriousness of his chronic lung disease, which would be a clinical problem throughout his hospitalization. On the twelfth post-operative day, reporters were told that half of them would have to leave; as far as the hospital was concerned the media party was over.

The next day a valve broke in Barney Clark's implanted heart, and the reporters refused to leave. However interviews with the surgical team became almost impossible. Nevertheless pressure grew to provide positive news about the patient who had been front page news for many days. At some time in January or February, 1983, a reporter from the Salt Lake City public television channel managed to undertake two separate videotape interviews with Barney Clark. During these interviews the confused patient did not look well, and had nothing good to say about his venture. These videotapes were never publicly released or acknowledged to the press. In a later interview, in March, the Utah team selected the best vignette after apparently probing for more than half an hour to obtain a positive response from Barney Clark about the implant. The nation watched on national television as DeVries asked his patient who looked enfeebled and ashen faced, 'You got any words of advice for somebody that's going through this again?' Clark replied, 'Well, I'd tell them that it's worth it. If there's no alternative – they either die or they have it done' (Zinman 1983).

The selective withholding of information and the initial hype and unfounded claims of early clinical success set the media on a predictable and irrevocable course. Instead of a quiet, rigorous scientific assessment of this experimental technology, the involved parties attempted to gain approval for its use by promoting it publicly, through the media. In fact, the one agency that should have had jurisdiction over the experiment, the NIH, was eliminated from this role by a quirk of the American legal/medical system. The NIH was the primary funding agency for research on the artificial heart, including the work at Utah. But the Utah investigators sensed a growing disillusionment with the total artificial heart at the NIH as the federal agency was shifting its focus and giving grants to 'partial' or 'assist' devices. The Utah group, fearing a cutback in funding and a loss of momentum, decided to break from the NIH and continue development alone. The bold stroke by which they did this, only possible using the peculiarities of the American system, was to license production of the Jarvik–7 heart to a private company which would manufacture the heart formed by the University of Utah investigators. As a result of this move the NIH had no control over the actual physical product – the heart itself. Only the federal Food and Drug Administration (FDA) could rule on the clinical use of the product, and despite vigorous pleas from the NIH to refuse permission, the FDA submitted to the finding of the Utah IRB that the implantation of the artificial heart in humans was ethically acceptable. Thus the Utah team was effectively able to circumvent all governmental oversight or control over the experiment (Preston 1988, pp. 108–15).

COMMERCIAL PRESSURES AND THE ARTIFICIAL HEART

After the long drawn-out and negative clinical experience with Barney Clark, the University of Utah IRB insisted on closer scrutiny of further heart implants on a case by case basis. Dr DeVries became more and more vexed with the delays and made clear his intention to leave for a more hospitable environment if he was not given the opportunity to pursue his programme of more implantations. Officials at the Humana Heart Institute, in Louisville, Kentucky, pursued DeVries as ardently as American university coaches recruit outstanding high school athletes, and in effect they offered him a free hand to undertake his research. Humana officials arranged for DeVries to have a private practice which would triple his income (*Time* 1984). The lifeline of the artificial heart was apparently now connected directly to corporate headquarters.

On July 3, 1984, DeVries applied to the Humana Institutional Review Board in Louisville, a formality required by the move. Four weeks later, he announced his intention to move to Louisville, which he did before the Humana IRB gave official approval on September 10, 1984. The unanimous decision of the sixteen member board to allow the surgical team to proceed with the six more implants already allowed by the FDA was in remarkable contrast to the deliberations and divisions of the Utah IRB. The Humana IRB had no experience in dealing with this sort of issue, and when interviewed later, some members did not know that they had made a different decision than that of the Utah IRB. DeVries's move before the official approval of the IRB had been granted from a body which was itself constituted by members who had an interest in promoting Humana, naturally raised the question among observers as to whether the Humana IRB had merely acted as a rubber stamp to a decision that had already been taken (Preston 1988 p. 124)

Spokespersons for the Humana Heart Institute denied that profit-making acted as an incentive for the arrangement with the team led by Dr DeVries. President Wendell Cherry defended the use of the plastic heart with an ironic metaphor, 'My heart is as ethical as any-one's heart.' Chairman Jones said they were doing it to gain 'prestige' within the medical community, and, as he was widely quoted, 'We hope to establish Humana as a brand name that stands for high-quality health care services at affordable prices' (Preston 1988 p. 124). The free media coverage Humana received from its first implant was probably worth more than millions of dollars of paid television advertising. As *Business Week* pointed out after Humana's first implant, the number of those enrolled in the chain's health maintenance organization more than doubled in the next six months. They con-cluded: 'Jones' shrewdest move to date – attracting the celebrated DeVries to Humana – has already paid off in spades' (*Business Week* 1985).

Proponents say major commercial involvement in the development of technology is necessary to infuse much needed capital into projects too large to be undertaken by non-profit research institutions. They point to the value of 'risk taking', the enhancement of innovation, and the speedier marketing of beneficial medical products. Of the principals in the Utah experiment to whom I broached the subject of a possible conflict of interest with their connection to the for-profit company making the artificial hearts (in which the head surgeon held a sizeable interest), only one, a social worker, expressed concern. As is well known, this sort of relationship between researchers and commercial funders of technology is standard procedure in the United States. Nevertheless, many of the leading figures in American medi-cine have doubts about this situation. They fear that precious resources will be diverted from basic research to more profitable lines of work, in the end to the detriment of other legitimate interests in society. Dr Arnold Relman, past editor of the *New England Journal of Medicine*, has decried Humana's excessive interest in publicity, noting 'Whatever they invest in paying for hospital care they certainly expect to gain back many times over. It's just like a commercial organization promoting the release of a new product' (Grady 1983). The fear expressed in this view, whether from elitism or insight, is that commercial co-opting of medical research will undermine the entire medical research structure, producing expensive therapies of limited value instead of fundamental medical advances. With regard to the artificial heart, the weight of capital seeking a saleable product is almost certain to produce a course of development different from the originally planned progression of the artificial heart programme. The introduction of strong commercial pressures into the artificial heart programme creates the risk of premature dissemination of a device that may be harmful to its recipients and could lead to public disillusionment and rejection of the entire programme.

WHO CHOOSES MEDICAL TECHNOLOGY?

The central issue which arises out of this discussion is whether the development and use of the artificial heart should be directed by a small group of medical investigators and those who are backing them with entrepreneurial funds and interests, or should be directed by the representatives of the society at large which has developed the technology and those who will have to live with its consequences. It appears to be a classic conflict between the economic independence and liberty of individuals to pursue their aims, and the public good, set in the context of an increasingly interdependent society. Resolution of the many political and ethical issues surrounding the artificial heart will not be possible until the central issue of who makes policy in relation to major technological developments is decided.

The fundamental issue is one of public involvement in the decision to continue the policy of artificial heart implantation. Until now policy has been formulated by a relatively small group of federal policy-makers; the physicians and engineers involved in the research and development of the artificial heart programme, and the representatives of private enterprise involved in its development. The government has failed to provide a meaningful assessment of the technology, or provide a clear lead in the development of policy. In 1988 Claude Lenfant, the NIH director in charge of the artificial heart programme, announced he was suspending funding for the total artificial heart, in favour of funding for partial assist devices. This brought an outcry from artificial heart manufacturers and investigators, and ultimately political considerations overrode a rational research decision. The contractors who stood to lose from the cessation of funding enlisted powerful political support which led to pressure on the NIH. Claude Lenfant's superiors ordered him to rescind his suspension of funding (Gil 1989 pp. 24–31).

The overriding point in this analysis is that a federal policy involving the expenditure of billions of dollars should not be directed almost exclusively by physicians and technicians who themselves have personal stakes in the policy, or by some politicians who promote special interests, but should be directed by more broadly based representatives of the public at large. Policy on such issues with all their ramifications, not the least of which are their social consequences, should be established by the Congress of the United States, following impartial scientific assessment of the relevant technology. The control of the development and use of major medical technology requires decision-making at the highest public level, for such technology has consequences for everyone.

MIRACLE MEDICINE

An important spin-off from the publicity attached to the development of the artificial heart, but not at all unique to that technology, is the reinforcement of the public predilection for a modern style of miracle medicine. The history of medicine is replete with the enthusiastic introduction of remedies, surgical procedures, and devices promoted by physicians and eagerly sought by a receptive public. All but a very few have been slowly and quietly abandoned, replaced by the next 'cure'. The public and professional avidity for promised cures is based on an important component of therapy: hope nurtured by excitement. The modern manifestation of traditional medicine with its associated symbols and rituals is complex technology, and the artificial heart is now on the leading edge of such technology. By allowing the Barney Clark experiment to become primarily a media event, with the main focus on the human story surrounding the recipient, the Utah team reinforced the public search for miracles. Further, the actions of the team deflected efforts from the more important business of educating everyone to the hard choices that must be made, either by them or their representatives, or by those medical authorities concerned with research and clinical practice. The existence of the artificial heart with its perceived potential for benefit, and the public pressure for such a new technology, appear to force decisions to be made that are not based for the most part on formal medical and research evaluation, but on clear social and political grounds. How the issue of the artificial heart is publicly managed will influence the lives of everyone much more than the few years of added corporeal existence the device may provide for some people. The stakes in relation to such technological developments are too high, and their consequences too great, to make relevant decisions without the fullest public scrutiny.

REFERENCES

Bernstein, B.J. (1984), 'The misguided quest for the artificial heart', *Technology Review*, November/December, p. 62

Business Week (1985), 'Humana: making the most of its place in the spotlight', May 6, pp. 68–9

Gil, G. (1989), 'The artificial heart juggernaut', *Hastings Centre Report*, March/April, pp. 24–31

Grady, D. (1983), 'Artificial heart skips a beat', *Medical Month*, December, p. 44

Jarvik, R. K. (1981), 'The total artificial heart', *Scientific American*, CCIVIV, p. 77

National Heart, Lung and Blood Institute (1973), *The Totally Implantable Artificial Heart*, DHEW Publication No. (NIH) 74–191, Bethesda, Maryland, June, pp. 14–16

Preston, T. A. (1983), 'The case against the artificial heart', *Seattle Weekly*, March 30, p. 25

—— (1985), 'Who benefits from the artificial heart?', *The Hastings Centre Report*, February, pp. 5–7

—— (1988), 'The artificial heart', in D. B. Dutton (ed.), *Worse Than The Disease*, Cambridge University Press, pp. 91–126

Time, (1984), 'Earning profits, saving lives', December 10, p. 85

Zinman, D. (1983), 'Improving the artificial heart', *Newsday*, August 1

8

Biotechnology, patients and profits: how is the law to respond?

MICHAEL FREEMAN

Biotechnology has become big business, but as yet legislatures and courts have had little opportunity to respond. The responses thus far have been tentative, fumbling, even incoherent. But I believe an examination of one of these, the Californian Supreme Court decision in *Moore* v *Regents of The University of California* (793 P. 2d 479 Cal. 1990) is instructive. This paper is an examination of the Court's reasoning and its deficiencies and an attempt to argue that the answer may lie in the development of a property right, or quasi-property right.

The question raised in the *Moore* case is 'If a patient's tissues are used as source material for the commercial development of high technology products, what property rights can the patient assert over his cells and the profit generated from the sale of those products' (Howard 1989 p. 333)? Previously, in 1980, the US Supreme Court had held (447 US 1980 p. 303) that patient protection extended to genetically engineered bacteria: 'A live, human-made micro organism . . . is patentable subject – matter' (447 US 1980 p. 305,310) said the Court in *Diamond* v *Chakrobarty*. Rosenberg, writing in *Clinical Research*,[1] responded that 'the biotechnology revolution ha[d] moved . . . from the classroom to the boardroom and from the *New England Journal [of Medicine]* to the *Wall Street Journal*'.

Since the *Diamond* case, biotechnology has attracted massive investments and become a highly commercial industry. The universities have not been left out of the race to exploit this new and highly-profitable market.

Biotechnology research on human cells consists broadly of three technologies: (i) tissue and cell culture technology; (ii) hybridoma technology; and (iii) recombinant DNA technology. The promise of these methods is the development of new drugs and treatments which may alter conventional medical practice. The commercial value of these developments cannot be readily calculated but, as an example, an estimate of the products from John Moore's cell line based on his leukaemia cell was 3 billion dollars by the year 1990.

Biotechnology has altered the practices of the medical research community. It has also had an incalculable impact on the relationship between doctors and researchers and patients. Clearly, when physicians are also researchers whose work on the patient can lead to financial profit, the latter may take priority, or at least it runs the risk of seeming to conflict with duties towards patients. The doctor who engages in biotechnological research uses as 'raw material' his patient's tissue and may develop commercial and profitable biotechnology products from this. This may, it hardly needs saying, lead to compromise over the patient's best medical treatment to promote personal and commercial interests. For example, the doctor may go beyond what is strictly necessary for treatment to obtain, or gain easier access to, material for experimentation and commercial exploitation.

This dilemma has found a partial answer in the development of the doctrine of informed consent[2] to include disclosure by the doctor-researcher of any personal, academic or commercial interest in the patient's cells, or the specific treatment recommended. Thus, in soliciting the patient's consent to treatment or removal of tissues, the doctor has to disclose any potential or other economic gain that he or she (or anyone else, so far as they know) may obtain from the post-operative use of the patient's tissues. Without such disclosure, any consent received would not be an 'informed' or valid one. In addition, the doctor would be in breach of his fiduciary duty.

However these are not my concerns here. The *Moore* case raises the possibility of the recognition of a property right over cells and other tissue. Should the law recognise human tissue as the personal property of the individual from whom it derives? Should the law permit the individual to sell his or her tissue? These are questions of deep moral significance. The *Moore* court failed to meet the challenge. We must look at its reasoning and see why. It is an issue which will not go away, and other courts and other institutions are bound to be confronted with claims such as that made by John Moore.

It all started in 1976 when Moore learned that he had hairy cell leukaemia. He approached the Medical Center of the University of California at Los Angeles. Under the supervision of Dr David Golde, the doctor who had attended Moore at UCLA, he was hospitalised and went through a series of tests which included the withdrawal of extensive amounts of blood and cells. It is the case that at the time all five defendants were aware of the great commercial and scientific value of Moore's cells.[3] On Dr Golde's recommendation of treatment, Moore signed a written consent form, authorising the removal of his spleen. Before the spleen was removed Golde had already given instructions that removed spleen cells were to be transferred to separate research units. These research activities had no relation to Moore's medical care. He was not told: his permission was not sought. In the next seven years Moore returned several more times to the UCLA Medical Center because he was told this was medically necessary. In fact, on each visit, Golde withdrew additional samples of blood, skin, bone-marrow and sperm. It is assumed[4] that throughout Golde and the Medical Center were engaged in extensive research on Moore's cells and planning their commercial exploitation. In short, this commercial exploitation included establishing an immortal cell line from Moore's T- lymphocytes, applying and securing a patent on the cell line, and entering with other defendants[5] into the development and manufacture of important therapeutic drugs. Dr. Golde and his research assistant were named as the inventors of these drugs. Moore never challenged the decision to remove his spleen: it may have saved his life. But he attempted to state 13 causes of action including

1 conversion
2 lack of informed consent
3 breach of fiduciary duty
4 fraud and deceit
5 unjust enrichment.

The Court of Appeal for the Second District of California (reversing a lower court) held that a person has a tangible property right in his or her own tissues, and that conversion occurs when these bodily constituents are taken for any purpose without the patient's consent.[6] The Court reasoned that, since a person has the ultimate right to control his or her own body, commercialisation of a patient's tissues by a doctor without prior consent could give rise to an action for damages.

The defendants' appeal was heard by an *en banc* Supreme Court of California. It considered only three of Moore's causes of action: conversion; breach of fiduciary duty, and lack of informed consent. As to the conversion claim, the majority (five judges) held that a cell line could not be a patient's 'property', so that the conversion cause of action had to fail. The Court agreed that the claims as to breach of fiduciary duty and lack of informed consent did disclose causes of action. The majority purports to show that Moore could achieve what he wanted under the latter causes of action. But it is on the decision as to property rights that I will concentrate. The reasoning is poor, often incoherent, and it fails to live up to the challenge of biotechnology. Only the dissenting opinion of Mosk J does in any way meet this challenge.

The essence of the property issue was put like this by the Court (793 P. 2d p. 487 Cal. 1990). It characterises conversion as 'a tort that protects against interference with possessory and ownership interests in personal property', and says that Moore 'theorizes that he continued to own his cells following their removal from his body, at least for the purpose of directing their use, and that he never consented to their use in potentially lucrative medical research', and that he claims 'A proprietary interest in each of the products that any of the defendants might ever create from his cells or the patented cell line.'

In the majority opinion (of Panelli J) Moore's allegation was examined under the existing law and found wanting (793 P. 2d 489–90). No reported common law decision could be found which recognised human cells as capable of being the subject of property and of being converted. This is not quite true since it passes over *Doodeward* v *Spence* (1908 6 CLR 406). It is an old Australian authority, not strictly on the point (it relates to trouver of an unburied human corpse) and it is confusing and unsatisfactory. It went on to state several problems with the idea of ownership of cells. Moore relied *inter alia* on the opinion of US courts that every person has a proprietary interest in his or her own likeness,[7] and alleged that 'if the courts have found a sufficiently proprietary interest in one's persona how could one not have a right in one's own genetic material, something far more profoundly the essence of one's human uniqueness than a name or a face?' (793 P. 2d p. 490 Cal. 1990).

The Court's unsatisfactory response was that lymphokines 'have the same molecular structure in every human being and the same important functions in every human being's immune system' (793 P. 2d p. 490 Cal. 1990). Moreover, said the Court, the particular genetic material which is responsible for the natural production of lymphokines, and which the defendants used in the manufacturing process is 'also the same in every person; it is no more unique to Moore than the number of vertebrae in the spine or the chemical formula of haemoglobin' (793 P. 2d p. 490 Cal. 1990).

This cannot be sustained: it surely is irrelevant to the tort of conversion that what is converted is to be found everywhere. Property is based on a relationship between a person and an object: that the object is one of a class commonly or even universally found is alien to the theory of property rights. Of course, if Moore's cells were really like everyone else's, they would not have been exploited for profit. The fact that the genes, though similar in every human being cell, were arranged in a way which has value for the researchers makes them unique, not in their essence but in their ability to be easily located. The anomalous nature of the Court's reasoning can be demonstrated by imagining that Moore's spleen had been given to him in a formalin jar. It could not then be unlawfully removed by the doctors, or anyone else.

The Court also relied on legislation[8] dealing with the disposal of unwanted or used human tissue to dismiss Moore's claim of ownership. The practical effect of this legislation, said the Court, is 'to limit, drastically, a patient's control over excised cells. By restricting how excised cells may be used and requiring their eventual destruction, the statute eliminates so many of the rights ordinarily attached to property that one cannot simply assume that what is left amounts to 'property' or 'ownership' for purposes of conversion law' (793 P. 2d p. 492 Cal. 1990). But this reasoning will not do. The statute referred to tackles matters of public hygiene and to do this it limits rights. It circumvents what a person may do with what is his or hers. But it is no less 'his' or 'hers' because they cannot do with it what they wish. Implicit in the Court's reasoning is the assumption that ownership is absolute or it is not ownership. That this is wrong hardly needs demonstration. If correct it would make much twentieth century social legislation (rent acts, for example) confiscatory. Furthermore, what the Court ignored is that the effect of the statute and its limitation would only take effect after the cells have been lawfully transferred to the researchers and the use of them has terminated. The statute is of no relevance at all to the transaction before material becomes waste. In any case, it does not indicate that a doctor who removes a patient's cells has a greater right to dispose than the patient himself.

The Court refused to recognise Moore's property in the patent (the patented cell line and the products derived from it) because the patented cell line is 'factually and legally distinct from the cells taken from Moore's body' (793 P. 2d p. 492). The Court asserted that what is protected by law is the patenting of organisms that represent the product of 'human ingenuity' but not 'naturally occurring organisms' (793 P. 2d p. 492 Cal. 1990). But this argument will not stand up either. Factually, the cells in the cell line are identical to the cells in Moore's body. The patent was granted for the success in establishing an immortal cell culture, but the components of the culture remained the same as Moore's cells and are in no way 'factually and legally distinct'. What the Court also seems to miss in this argument is that Moore was not claiming ownership over the patent, but over the cell line, namely over his cells multiplying and thriving in the laboratory. In addition, Moore pointed out that, without his cells as raw material, no cell line (incidentally called Mo cell line after him) could have been established. He, therefore, claimed a share in the establishment of the cell line. Of course, if most of the value of the patent is the result of the efforts of the researchers, then the share of the profits to which Moore would be entitled for contributing the raw material would be limited. The grant of the patent over the invention of the cell line has nothing to do with Moore's claim of conversion of his cells. The cells themselves are not the subject-matter of the patent and could never be so. Accordingly, the existence of the patent is no answer to the allegation of conversion.

Moore's claim thus, in the opinion of the majority, failed under the existing law. But could the existing law be expanded? The Court gave three reasons why they were unprepared to this. First, 'a fair balancing of the relevant policy considerations counsels against extending the tort' (793 P. 2d p. 493 Cal. 1990). Secondly, the area of development was better suited to legislative resolution. And, thirdly, the tort of conversion was 'not necessary' (793 P. 2d p. 493 Cal. 1990) to protect patients' rights. The first two of these reasons do not survive critical scrutiny. The Court saw two policy considerations: (i) protection of a competent patient's right to make autonomous medical decisions; and (ii) protection against 'disabling civil liability' (793 P. 2d p. 493 Cal. 1990) of 'innocent third parties ... engaged in socially useful activities, such as researchers who have no reason to believe that their use of a particular cell sample is, or may be, against a donor's wishes'. They had to be balanced and the outcome of this balance, in the Court's view, was 'liability based upon existing disclosure obligations rather than an unprecedented extension of the conversion theory'. This would, the Court believed, protect 'patients' rights of privacy and autonomy without unnecessarily hindering research' (793 P. 2d p. 494 Cal. 1990). But is this right?

First, it seems the Court has identified the patient's interest which needs protection wrongly. It is not his right of privacy that should have concerned the Court: rather his right to property in his cells. But, having done this, the Court was led into trying to find a way of protecting privacy (without hindering research) and it found this in informed consent. This caused it to deviate from the central issue which is whether conversion can be applied to the unauthorised dealing with a person's cells. Even if the informed consent theory were sufficient to protect the patient's interest, it is difficult to see how it can allow or justify the commercial exploitation of that patient's cells

Secondly, not content with a misplaced identification of interests, the Court got the balancing wrong as well. It was concerned lest an extension of the tort of conversion might jeopardise biotechnological research. 'The extension of conversion law into this area will hinder research by restricting access to the necessary raw materials.' The Court pointed to the many diseases (leukaemia, cancer, diabetes, hepatitis-B etc.) for which treatments and tests have been developed as a result of developments within biotechnology. But why should human 'raw material' be different from other products used in research? If the researcher wants to do experiments on animals he or she has to purchase animals or their tissue. Why should human products such as cells be different? Big profits are being made. Why should not the person from whom the raw material emanates have his or her share too? The Court's concern to protect big business against the 'little man', for it can be so characterised, would be difficult to fathom if it were not so common.

If we turn to the Court's second reason (the view that legislation is best left to the legislature), we are on familiar ground, It is a respectable view. But does it hold here? What was the Court being asked to do? It was not being asked to create a new field of law, a new tort, for example. It was being asked to apply (extend, if you prefer it) existing doctrine to a new set of circumstances. The dissenting judge (Mosk J) was surely right when, quoting *Rodriguez* v *Bethlehem Steel Corp*(1974 12 Cal. 3rd p. 382, 394), he said (793 P. 2d p. 507 Cal. 1990), 'Although the legislature may of course speak to the subject, in the common law system the primary instruments of this evolution are the courts, adjudicating on a regular basis the rich variety of individual cases brought before them.'

A number of other points may be made about the Court's reasoning and its implications. The Court contented itself that it could do justice by a holding in breach of fiduciary duty. But this is an unsatisfactory conclusion. First, because it does not tackle the question of property at all. Secondly, because it only protects, insofar as it protects at all, against those who are in a relationship with the patient. Mosk J, in his dissent, hypothesises thus. Suppose 'another medical center or a drug manufacturer stole the cells after removal and used them in an unauthorized manner for its own economic gain' (793 P. 2d p. 521 Cal. 1990). Since there would clearly be no breach of fiduciary duty, the patient would have to vindicate his or her rights in a conversion action. Thirdly, to prove breach of fiduciary duty is difficult. The patient will have to prove that if he or she had been informed of the commercial value of the operation and of his cells, they would have declined their consent (or perhaps, any reasonably prudent patient would). But in reality few, if any, would decline. It is likely that, at the very least, the patient would be influenced by medical advice that the removal of an enlarged spleen would save or at least prolong his or her life. Fourthly, although we could, and perhaps should, extend the scope of fiduciary duty, at the moment it is accepted that it applies to pre-existing interests only. The doctor does not have to disclose his or her future research interests or the commercial possibilities associated with the medical intervention. This is not consistent with the autonomy notion which is the basis of the informed consent doctrine.

Finally, the reasoning of the majority in *Moore* leaves us with a strange conclusion. Moore cannot benefit from the Mo cell line, but Dr Golde and the other defendants who obtained Moore's cells without his consent are the lawful owners of those cells and the patent in the cell line and can exploit the full economic value of them. Indeed, if John Moore were to enter the laboratories at the University of California and re-take his cells, he would be civilly liable for the tort of conversion and criminally liable in theft.

A strange conclusion reached, it may be thought, by strange and unsatisfactory reasoning. We must therefore leave the decision as such and consider the ethical arguments that may be used to support, or indeed to deny, John Moore's claim.

The Court was clearly influenced by such utilitarian considerations as scientific advance and better medical solutions. In addition it is common knowledge that funding for research is likely to be more readily forthcoming if tangible benefit in its outcome can be guaranteed by law. There is a critical equation here, but the Court only saw one side of it. It ignored the fact that prospective donors of raw material will be more likely to come forward if offered the incentive to participate in the profit. As Danforth put it,[9]

> research with human cells that results in significant economic gain for the researchers and no gain for the patient offends the traditional morals of our society in a manner impossible to quantify . . . The dignity and sanctity with which we regard the whole human body, as well as mind and soul, are absent when we allow researchers to further their own interests without the patient's participation by using a patient's cells as a basis for a marketable product.

If scientific progress is so all-important a consideration, then why allow anyone to have property rights in a cell line, for example? Free movement of scientific resources may be even more beneficial to mankind than the protection of the property rights of the original researcher. But it may not, and experience tells us (at least within capitalism) that scientific progress is more likely when there is the lure of profit.

So it seems that research must be rewarded. However, recognising property rights in our own cells accords with our concept of fairness and justice. The notion that the person whose cells bring profit to others is him- or herself neglected is not consonant with our intuitive ideas of fairness and justice. This conclusion obtains support also from a comparison with that reached in other areas. Rare cases apart, the law prohibits the exploitation or any use by one person of a thing which does not belong to him: if such a thing is illegally used a share of the profit is due to the person whose property it is. Some qualms may be felt about selling blood or semen (rather than donating it), but this is done. People do profit by using their body for commercial purposes.

The majority in the *Moore* case discussed at length the implications, as they saw them, of recognising a property interest in one's bodily tissues. Six interests at least come into play. They are:

(1) the interest of the person from whom the tissues come to self-determination (including obtaining value from his cells)

(2) his interests to be treated professionally, to possess full knowledge of the implications of his treatment in order to make decisions which further his best interests

(3) the interest of society that new treatments and medicines are developed and that research towards the elimination or amelioration of disease is accelerated

(4) the researcher's interest in scientific achievement and personal gain (including financial benefit)

(5) the interest of the pharmaceutical industry to obtain new 'raw material', to maximise its profits and to finance further research

(6) the societal interest in obviating unwanted side effects attendant upon the recognition of property rights, such as the patient's decision being based upon commercial considerations rather than strictly medical, therapeutic or altruistic ones.

Doubtless other interests can also be identified. It is easy to separate the interests, to atomise almost, but in reality they can be combined. Society needs new remedies for acute diseases: it also needs people to be willing to participate. We cannot, nor, I would add, should we, assume that such participation can be secured by altruistic motives alone. Incentives may be necessary. If potential participants feel they are going to be exploited, as Moore, for example, claims he was, their willingness to co-operate may diminish. The right balance (for balance is what we are ultimately seeking) between the interests identified above may be to recognise at least a limited property right in one's tissues. Such recognition will affirm individual autonomy and self-determination whilst assisting research, helping the biotechnology industry to profit and promoting the maximisation of the societal interest in scientific progress and medical advance.

We must look at the issue of property rights from the perspective of the doctor-patient relationship. Tissue may come from healthy donors, but it is more likely to emanate from patients, since the most needed tissues in biotechnological research are rare pathological ones.[10] Moreover, in most cases the discovery of the rare cell or particularly valuable gene occurs by chance during regular or routine tests on the already-hospitalised patient.[11] The patient is likely to vest enormous trust in those treating him or her. It should, therefore, be a firm rule, as Howard puts it (1989 p. 339) that 'physician recommendations about the patient's diagnostic and treatment options should be based solely on the patient's interest in health, not on the physician's interest in maximising the commercial possibilities of the patient's tissues'.

Modern techniques of research and the use of genetic bio- engineering make it much easier for doctors and researchers to acquire the human raw data they seek, using the samples given by the trusting patient at a preliminary test. This reduces what little power patients may have to bargain and protect their interests. Property rights in human cells would reduce this imbalance, and assist a process which could recognise the interests of both doctors and patients.

The 'autonomy factor' should also not be ignored. Everyone has a basic right to autonomy and privacy, a right to determine the use of his or her body. That much is uncontentious or relatively so. In the *Moore* case[12] the court did recognise that 'a patient must have the ultimate power to control what becomes of his or her tissues. To hold otherwise would open the door to a massive invasion of human privacy and dignity in the name of medical progress'. But the Court, driven by fear of, what it considered to be, the effect of recognising property rights in human tissue, went on to assert[13] that it is possible 'to protect privacy and dignity without accepting the extremely problematic conclusion that interference with those interests amounts to a conversion of personal property... The fiduciary duty and informed consent theories protect these interests directly by requiring full disclosure.'

But, whilst the informed consent doctrine is based on autonomy and self-determination rights,[14] it cannot provide a total answer. It can, for example, not give any right to nonpatient donors. The British Human Tissue Act (and its American parallel)[15] recognises that no individual has the power to decide what should be done with his corpse after death. If autonomy can be exercised in this way, why not, it may be argued, also during the individual's lifetime.

This is the case for the recognition of property rights in one's cells. It is, I believe, a substantial one, but the arguments the other way must not be overlooked. They are threefold. First, recognition of property rights in the human body would eventually lead to the commodification of the human body. Secondly, sharing the profits of biotechnological research would increase the expenses of the research and of the production of the final drugs or treatment. This would result in more expensive medicine for the sick. A similar argument is that giving the patients the right to demand money for their participation would bring 'a bidding war between companies for rare tissues' and 'could significantly increase the cost of tissue' (O'Connor 1990 p. 149). Thirdly, it may lead to patients adopting new priorities, placing their financial well-being ahead of their health or welfare. Patients may be tempted, or indeed enticed, to choose a treatment not by its effectiveness but by the lure of financial profit.

Each of these objections must be critically examined. As to the first, the fears are clear and genuine. There is real concern of a trade in human organs, with the poor not being able to buy and other poor people being tempted (or coerced) into selling semi-essential organs like kidneys. We have experienced the latter recently with the revelation of Turkish peasants being exploited by allegedly reputable London surgeons. But this is not what is in issue in the 'cells' debate. It is, it is submitted, rather different if for no other reason than that cells are regenerative. This distinction is recognised in the recent Human Organs Transplants Act 1989, which makes it an offence to trade, or offer to trade, in any way, in living or dead human organs for transplantation. The Act defines 'organ'[16] as a 'structured arrangement of tissues which, if wholly removed, cannot be replicated by the body'. Cells are thus left out of the application of this Act. There is also a distinction between organs reserved solely for the purpose of transplantation and those removed, as in the case of Moore's spleen, as a part of therapeutic treatment. But, ultimately, where the commodification objection fails is in identifying what the objection is: 'While moral aversion to pricing the human body may argue against biotechnology as a whole, as long as commercial exploitation of the body continues, the argument should not deny profit participation to the patient alone' (Hardiman 1986 p. 240). Unless we are prepared to ban biotechnology, we should not use our discomfort with it to penalise the 'victim' of it.

The second objection may well have validity but not enough to reject the right of the patient to a share in the profits produced from his tissues. It is true that the costs of investment in any biotechnological product are enormous (an official US report put it at between 65 and loo million dollars per product).[17] And, it is reckoned that only 12 per cent of the products which enter clinical trials ever get as far as the market. The *Moore* court gave priority to these arguments.[18] But researchers pay for guinea pigs, equipment and staff and pay other companies for their property (drugs, chemicals, etc.). Indeed, there are special payments for rare laboratory animals. Should all these be given free of charge to facilitate biotechnological research? It is sometimes argued in addition that if there is to be reimbursement there will be negotiation and this will cause delay (O'Connor 1990 p. 129). But if this incident of capitalism is unacceptable, it could be removed by regulation (for example, a fixed method of payment such as a percentage).

The third objection is a weighty one and has to be addressed. The combination of distress and poverty and the opportunity to acquire security for self or family may indeed attract persons to put financial above medical considerations. The Hippocratic oath should act as a barrier to prevent this happening (Beauchamp and Childress 1989

p. 120), but some doctors will abuse their power and betray the trust of their patients, and some have done so. Indeed, as pressure and competition become greater, and the race for achievement tougher, some doctors may lack the power to resist the temptation to put their scientific goals before their patients' welfare. These are problems to be acknowledged and to be addressed. The importance of ethical committees in tackling them is crucial. But nothing is foolproof and the unscrupulous will occasionally fall through the net. This does not, however, convince that all patients should lose out because a few do not put their best (or what we consider to be their best) interests first.

The conclusion reached is that a property right in one's cells ought to be recognised, that the arguments adduced to deny it on Moore are unsound and unsatisfactory, and the ethical arguments in favour of such a right are persuasive and the fears of objectors exaggerated. If this conclusion is acceptable, a further question must be addressed. On what principle is the commercial interest to be realised? Briefly, there are four models:

1 Free market negotiation
2 A fixed price (a 'flat fee basis')[19]
3 A percentage of the profits, said by one supporter (Noonan)[20] to eliminate the ghoulish necessity of bargaining with patients over their cells and providing 'reasonable compensation to the source of their tissue'.
4 A share of the profits or the so-called 'right of commerciality' (Hardiman 1986 p. 258).

Although the case put in this chapter has been for the property rights of the patient, the interests of society and of science have not been overlooked. The balancing equation means that the property interest must be a limited one and this consideration alone would rule out the first model. But it can be excluded for other reasons: the familiar, well-rehearsed arguments about the inequalities of bargaining power and distortions in decision-making abilities.

The fixed price model may be difficult to operationalise because of the difficulties of predicting the true potential of the tissues. A fixed fee system could well lead to later litigation when the true profit became known.

It is therefore to the latter two models that I turn. There is not a lot to distinguish them. The third model is, however, more rigid and for this reason I advocate the fourth. It got the blessing of the Californian Court of Appeals (202 Cal. App. 3rd 1230). The right to share would only arise when the body was exploited for profit. As Hardiman puts it: 'The right of commerciality would protect the value of one's body or its derivatives, prevent its misappropriation and the unjust enrichment of others, and place the individual in an equal bargaining position with researchers, medical institutes and biotechnology operations.'

The starting point is the recognition of property rights in human tissues, but the emphasis is on the property right in the commercial value of one's body rather than in the tissues themselves. The focus is on the profits, rather than the body itself. The right would only arise when the body is exploited for profit: only then could the individual involved demand compensation. The right of commerciality would only arise when there was any profit. Thus non-profit organisations would not be harmed, and the practice of donating organs voluntarily would not be affected.

This is, it is conceded, not without problems. Three, briefly, will be mentioned. First, profits are often a long time in coming. Would this lead to arguments many years after the removal of tissues? The patient might by then be dead. The possibility of litigation with his or her personal representatives cannot be overlooked. Secondly, the patient will lose out if the researcher or institution involved does not succeed in making any profit or drops the research or is beaten by competitors. The 'right of commerciality' in such circumstances amounts to very little. Thirdly, there is a case for paying the patient even when the profits are ultimately non-existent. The researcher pays for the guinea pig and staff irrespective of the end profit result. By participating in the project the patient is assisting the researcher in all sorts of ways: the research project will bring prestige, assist the gaining of research money and promote the institution. It may indirectly foster subsequent research.

The right of commerciality is a serious attempt to recognise the rights of persons to a share in the profits derived from the use of their cells. It does not, it has been seen, protect property rights in full. It could only do this if it were recognised as a full, unlimited property right. But this would fail to recognise the other interests involved. The right accordingly has to be limited (a 'quasi' property right' one commentator has called it (Hardiman 1986 p. 261)). We are only at the beginning of the path which will lead to legal remedies in this complex and sensitive area. This chapter has identified the issues and problems and postulated a tentative conclusion. Nothing more would be warranted presently.

NOTES

1. (1986), 'Using patient materials for product development: a dean's perspective', *Clinical Research*, XXXIII, pp. 452, 453. See also B. I. Rowland, (1986), 'legal implications of letter licenses for biotechnology', *High Technology Law Journal*, I, pp. 99, 100–2 (on a dispute between Hoffman La Roche and UCLA).

2. See, in relation to the *Moore* case, D. Daniels, (1990) 'Commercialization of human tissues: has biotechnology created the need for an expanded scope of informed consent?', *California Western Law Review*, XXXVII, p. 209; *Harvard Law Review* (1990), 'Recent developments: tort law-informed consent – California's Supreme Court recognises patient's cause of action for physician's non-disclosure of excised tissues' commercial value', CIV, p. 808; S. N. Perley, (1992), 'From control over one's body to control over one's body parts: extending the doctrine of informed consent', *New York University Law Review*, LXII, p. 335.

3. Moore's T-Lymphocyte blood cell has a unique nature in that it over-produced certain lymphokines. This quality made it easier to identify the gene responsible for the production of that type of lymphokine. In more standard cases the location of the relevant gene would be exceedingly difficult.

4. Certainly the Supreme Court of California assumed Moore's allegations to be true.

5. The defendants were Dr Golde, the physician who attended Moore at UCLA Medical Center, the Regents of the University of California, who own and operate the university, Shirley Quan, a researcher employed by the Regents, Genetics Institute Inc., and Sandoz Pharmaceuticals Corporation and related entities.

6. 202 Cal. App 3d. 1230, 1244–48. A critique of this is N. E. Field, (1989), 'Evolving conceptualizations of property: a proposal to de-commercialize the value of fetal tissue', *Yale Law Journal*, IC, p. 169.

7. *Lugosi* v. *Universal Pictures* (1929), 25 Cal. 3d 813; *Motschenbacher* v. *R. J.Reynolds Tobacco Co.* (19xx) 498 F. 2d 821. But in neither opinion did the court expressly base its holding on property law.

8. Health and Safety Code section 7054.4. p. 491.

9. See M. T. Danforth, (1988), 'Cells, sales and royalties: the patient's right to a portion of the profit', *Yale Law and the Policy Review* VI, pp. 179, 190. And see *Union Pacific Railway* v. *Botsford*, 141 US 250, 251 (1991): 'No right is held more sacred, or is more carefully guarded . . . than the right of every individual to the possession and control of her own person'.

10. See R. Freshney, *Culture of Animal Cells: A Manual of Basic Technique*, (2nd edn), p. 9.

11. Apparently only about 250 Americans a year contract hairy cell leukaemia and only a small percentage of them could be treated to establish a cell-line.

12. See J. J. O'Connor, (1990), 'The commercialization of human tissue, the source of legal, ethical and social problems: an area better suited to legislative resolution', *Loyola of Los Angeles Law Review*, XXIV, p. 115, 165. See, more generally, on autonomy R. Lindley, (1986), *Autonomy*, Macmillan, Basingstoke, and L. Haworth, (1986), *Autonomy*, Yale University Press, New Haven.

13. See W. D, Noonan, (1990) 'Ownership of biological tissues', *Journal of the Patent and Trademore Office Society*, LXXII, pp. 109, 111.

14. See P. S. Appelbaum, C. W. Lidz, A. Meisel, (1987), *Informed Consent: Theory and*

Clinical Practice, OUP pp. 22–31. See also S. A. M. McLean, (1989), *A Patient's Right To Know*, Dartmouth, Aldershot.

15. And see generally J. F. Blumstein, F. A. Sloan, (eds.), *Organ Transplantation Policy, Issues and Prospects,*

16. Human Organs Transplants Acts (UK) 1989, Section 7(2).

17. Office of Technology Assessment, US Congress, OTA, *New Developments In Biotechnology: Ownership of Human Tissues and Cells*, p. 61.

18. See 193 p. 2d pp. 487,493, Cal. 1990. 'The Court elevated social utility over individual rights' (see L. M. Ivey, (1991), 'Patients' rights in the biotechnological market', *Georgia Law Review*, XXV, pp. 489–519).

19. Once paid sources would relinquish all present and future rights in their tissues.

20. See Noonan 'Ownership of biological tissues'.

REFERENCES

Beauchamp, T. L., Childress, J. F. (1989), *Principles of Biomedical Ethics*, 3rd edn., OUP, p. 120

Hardiman, R. (1986), 'Towards the right of commerciality: recognising property rights in the commercial value of human tissue', *UCLA Law Review*, XXIV, pp. 207–240

Howard, J. J. (1989), 'Biotechnology, patients' rights and the Moore case', *Food, Drug and Cosmetic Law Journal*, XLIV, pp. 331–3

O'Connor, J. J. (1990), 'The commercialisation of human tissue, the source of legal, ethical, and social problems', *Loyola of Los Angeles Law Review*, XXIV, p. 115

9

A monopsonistic market: or how to buy and sell human organs, tissues and cells ethically

CHARLES A. ERIN AND JOHN HARRIS

Any system of commerce in human body parts and products presupposes that we hold property rights in those parts and products. In particular, for a commercial scheme to be properly predicated we must admit what Honoré terms 'the right to the capital', that is, 'the power to alienate the thing and the liberty to consume, waste or destroy the whole or part of it' (Honoré 1961 p. 118). An important point that seems often to be missed is that any system of voluntary donation of body parts and products seems also to presuppose ownership. In essence, whether we sell or donate or bequeath our organs and tissues, we must first own them. It is a heavy irony that when those who object to commerce in human biological materials say that profit should not figure in human organ procurement what they actually mean is the individual who supplies an organ should not profit – everyone else concerned profits.

The case of *Moore* v *The Regents of The University of California*[1] raises the question of whether individuals have full property rights in (that is own) biological materials obtained from their bodies. In ruling on the property element in the Moore case, the California Supreme Court decided against entertaining the concept of patients owning tissues removed at surgery.

The reasoning of the court in coming to this decision has been criticized for inconsistency and flawed argument (Scowen 1990), and it is not unlikely that when future, similar cases arise (and in our opinion they surely will) *Moore* will be found wanting as a precedent. We analyse here some possible consequences of an over-ruling of the decision on the property element in *Moore*, and take the proposition that individuals own organs, tissues and cells removed from their bodies as our starting premise.

Assigning ownership of the organs and tissues of her body to the individual opens the door to commerce in those organs and tissues in that it raises the presumption that the individual is entitled to dispose (in all senses of that term) of her property, a presumption which can, of course, be rebutted (for example consider the steward-ship of artworks, etc.) but which places the onus of justifying control on those who would seek to exercise it. Here we address this question: assuming we are to countenance commerce in human derived organs and tissues, of the various commercial schemes that may be pro-pounded which is to be preferred and how might it work?

Some initial distinctions may be drawn. Firstly we may distinguish between organs and tissues obtained from cadavers, and those obtained from living persons. Further, in the latter case (on which we concentrate here), distinguishing between the uses to which organs, tissues and cells are to be put may also prove helpful.

CADAVERS

Arguing for commerce in the context of organs obtained from cadavers is less morally problematic than in the case of the living. For a start, a cadaver cannot be argued, reasonably, to be a person and thus considerations of personal autonomy do not enter the picture: to talk of the autonomy of the dead is absurd. Each year several thousands of persons die prematurely from the lack of donated organs. Certain organs, hearts for example, can only be obtained from cadavers.[2] Whilst this shortfall of cadaver organs for transplantation persists it seems morally insupportable to ignore policies which would likely save lives unless they are counterbalanced by arguments of comparable moral force.

Such policies could include offering prospective payments for organs retrieved *post mortem*. Such prospective payments, whether in money or present medical care, are currently offered in some Ameri-can states in return for the delivery of one's body at death (Munzer 1990 p. 52). It has been argued that this would lead to a fall in the numbers of organs donated on purely humanitarian or altruistic grounds,[3] but nevertheless it seems probable that the introduction of such a commercial interest would lead to an overall increase in organ yield (Brams 1977; Buc and Bernstein 1984).

Alternatively legislation could be introduced placing cadaver organs in the public domain and hence authorising their compulsory removal where they will be used for life-saving transplantation (Harris 1992 pp. 102–3). In effect, where lives would be saved cadaver organs would automatically become public property. There is an analogy here with compulsory autopsies – the underlying rationale is the same: the perceived public interest. Is the saving of a life not arguably a better moral ground for the invasion of bodily integrity after death than curiosity about the cause of death?

Neither of these systems is unethical and the question of which is to be preferred is reduced to a question of practical efficacy. In terms of effectiveness, the case for the latter scheme is stronger, and stronger still if one considers the maximizing of health resources a priority.

LIVING PERSONS

We cannot apply similar reasoning to the procurement of organs and tissue from living people. Firstly, *compulsory* organ removal, even to save the life of another, violates the Kantian imperative against using persons solely as means to our ends and vitiates their autonomy. That is, we risk exploiting persons by using them merely as organ or tissue banks. This applies equally well to regenerative tissues as it does to non-regenerative tissues and vital organs. Secondly, unlike the dead, living persons are usually thought to have the right to freedom from physical violation which cannot be ignored. Furthermore, there may be an argument against conscription on general utilitarian grounds. For in psychological terms, rather than in terms of *realpolitik*, in so much as people fear the compulsory seizing of organs and tissues from the living, there seems to be no utility in enacting legislation which would establish a scheme of conscription.

EXPLOITATION

Our views on exploitation have been ventilated elsewhere (Harris 1992 Chapters 5 and 6; Erin and Harris 1991) and we will not rehearse our arguments in detail here. However, we note the main points as they relate to this issue so that the charge of exploitation commonly levelled at proposed commercial systems for the procurement of human organs, tissues and cells may be debunked.

Our treatment of others as a *means to our own ends* is a necessary condition for that treatment to constitute exploitation, but it is not a sufficient condition:

It is not wrong of itself to use people as means to our ends; what is wrong is using them merely or solely as means to our ends. The Kantian imperative lurking in the background here requires us to treat people as ends in themselves, as persons, and we can do this, and we do do this, when we invite them to adopt their capacity to help us, their contribution to ends of ours, as one of their own ends.
(Erin and Harris 1991 pp. 628–9)

Where we enlist others to act as means to our ends and they share those ends we are not truly exploiting them. Exploitation proper occurs when we treat them as means to our own ends *and* they do not make an autonomous decision to take on their part in our projects. In this situation they are subjected to some form of coercion against which they are vulnerable. Genuine exploitation must involve the violation of the autonomy of the exploited and we can try to make certain that our utilization of others is not a wrongful use by asking for their consent and respecting their option to withhold it.

Some believe that *paying* people to act as means to our ends is 'positively exploitative' (for example Warnock 1985 p. 46). If a person's acting as a means to our ends is exploitative, what difference can it make if they are paid to do so? It seems paradoxical that giving something away may be nonexploitative but being paid for the same thing may be exploitative. Is it that the mere fact of being offered money in some transaction necessarily erodes our autonomy? We submit that it is not, and that there must be shown to be some further element peculiar to the transaction for our autonomy to have been undermined by it. Thus, in the present context, it would need to be shown that there is something morally objectionable about the alienation of tissues independent of whether payment is involved (Harris 1992 Chapter 6). If it is not the very fact of payment that makes a transaction exploitative, could it be that it is the scale of payment which does so? That is to say, could it be that a transaction becomes exploitative when there is a disparity in the value of what is transferred and that of the payment received for it? The answer is that disparity in value *alone* does not make an exchange of goods or services wrongfully exploitative (Harris 1992).

PAYING OTHERS TO FACE DANGER

The living organ donor undertakes risks, risks which cannot be ascribed to a non-sentient cadaver. The risks of organ transplantation to the source arise from the use of anaesthesia, the surgery itself, and the possibility of post-operative complications. There are also the risks to the source's future health: for example, the individual who has undergone nephrectomy may herself require a kidney transplant in the future due to the failure of her remaining organ. Such risks tend to be exaggerated (Harris 1991) and are dwarfed by the risk to the organ recipient who may face imminent premature death if denied the requisite organ. Do we exploit others by paying them to undertake risks or face dangers on our behalf? This may appear implausible when we consider the many occupations (for example in the fire service) which involve occupational hazards. Again, however, whether paying people to take on risks for our ends constitutes exploitation will depend on other aspects of a certain transaction – whether the level of payment is inappropriate considering the *particular* risk or danger involved or whether they have been coerced into facing it.

EXPLOITATION OF POOR PEOPLE

With these general reflections on exploitation in mind we are in a position to consider a common and seemingly plausible criticism of any proposed market in bodily organs and tissues, that such a market would lead, necessarily, to exploitation of the poor. What is the basis of the charge? It might be thought that the choice to sell a body part in an attempt to better one's conditions becomes non-autonomous because one has no other option to this course of action than not to sell. But, *ceteris paribus*, we do not raise this objection to the poor selling other forms of property. It is likely that the objection is raised to the sale of body parts *per se*, especially organs, because this may result in the vendor being left in a disabled or somehow debilitated condition. However, this seems neither an adequate ground for the non-creation of a market nor for the exclusion of the poor from it. This attitude fails to take into account that for the poverty stricken mother, say, the sale of a body part, even if it does result in some form of disability, may present a more attractive option to not selling an organ and being unable to provide adequately for her children. We should compare this with the attitudes to the risk of occupational hazards, for example. Exploitation of the poor is, manifestly, morally objectionable, but we should not confuse our preventing their exploitation, however benevolent the motivation for such paternalism, with caring for or exercising moral obligations toward them. If we wish to show our concern for the poor, we should help them by alleviating their poverty.[4] Preventing them selling what little property they have seems a misguided way of doing this.

How are we to judge what price a particular live supplier of an organ should fetch on the market? There are undesirable effects linked to both over- and underpricing: set the price too high and there will be those in need of organs who cannot afford them; set the price too low and the system will be unlikely to attract vendors and a primary aim of establishing a market, to make up the shortfall in organ supply, will not be achieved. Furthermore, if prices are set too low the vendor could be said to be exploited; equally, if prices are set too high the purchaser could be said to be exploited.

This conception of exploitation thus implies that there exists a 'fair price' for a particular organ or tissue. How are we to decide what this price should be? In a free market we could perhaps leave it to market forces, but can we simply say that the going rate in a certain marketplace for a kidney or a cornea represents a fair price? In short, insofar as the idea of exploitation may be thought to presuppose some conception of a fair price, it seems clear that it would not be possible to arrive at a conception of a 'fair price' sufficiently plausible to sustain charges of exploitation.

THERAPY/RESEARCH

We are about to propose a possible commercial scheme, but first let us draw a distinction between human biological materials. For reasons which will become apparent below we divide these materials into two classes according to the use to which they are to be put: (i) those which are to be used for therapeutic purposes; and (ii) those which are to be utilized in research. In very general terms, this approximates to the distinction between organs and tissues/cells respectively. An organ is an aggregation of tissues constituting a structural unit with a particular function or functions. A tissue is a collection of cells, again with a specific function. Whilst John Moore's spleen was removed as part of his therapy for hairy cell leukaemia, it was the tissues and cells of his spleen which were used in the derivation of the Mo cell line (Erin 1994). However, blood, a fluid tissue, defies such a taxonomy as it is put to both therapeutic and research purposes.

ORGANS, TISSUES AND CELLS USED FOR THERAPY

Morally, the most desirable mode for obtaining sufficient human organs – and in general we are considering organs here – from living adults to meet the therapeutic need for them would be by donation. However, currently, and for the foreseeable future, this remains an ideal and we now consider how the existing shortfall in organs could be made up though the operation of a commercial scheme.

In devising a practical scheme we should be concerned to prevent morally objectionable exploitation. We use the phrase 'morally objectionable exploitation' here because we believe that in this context certain forms of exploitation involved in a transaction do not necessarily show such transactions in general to be morally objectionable. Thus, if it could be shown that in a particular transaction exploitation had occurred merely in as much as the vendor had been under-paid for her organ, this would not be a sufficient reason for a blanket suspension of commerce in organs – disputes over levels of payment could be resolved by, for example, arranging compensation. However, if the vendor's decision to sell was not an autonomous choice, we would then have a clear-cut case of morally objectionable exploitation, and such cases are to be avoided, even at the cost of a prospective organ recipient's life.

VULNERABLE PERSONS

The prevention of wrongful exploitation is not our only concern. We should also make provision for protection of vulnerable persons, and we should be careful not to confine the category of vulnerable persons to those liable to, or particularly liable to exploitation. We must not forget that in the kinds of transactions being discussed it is nearly always true to say that those in need of purchased organs (whom it is often tempting to label the exploiters in these exchanges) are at greater risk than the vendors. Without the purchased organ the prospective recipient may often stand to lose her life – and thus: 'There is a clear sense in which while would-be purchasers are necessarily vulnerable, would-be donors are only contingently so' (Harris 1992 p. 137). This category of vulnerable persons also demands our respect, and this is a consideration that should be taken into account when deciding on a pricing policy. Whilst an inappropriately low price may result in the exploitation of the vendor, an unaffordably high price could lead to the prospective purchaser's premature death.

A COMMERCIAL SCHEME: MONOPSONY

We now offer for consideration one possible commercial scheme which might work to make up the shortfall in live donor organs and tissues required for therapeutic purposes. Any such scheme must be morally defensible: it should have built into it safeguards against wrongful exploitation and show concern for vulnerable persons, as well as taking into account considerations of justice and equity.

One way of attending to this need for prudent regulation would be to establish a monopsony, that is 'a situation where only one buyer exists for the products of several sellers' (Schwarz *et al.* 1988). The one legitimate purchaser in the marketplace would be required to take on responsibility for ensuring equitable distribution of all organs and tissues purchased. This would prevent rich people using their purchasing power to exploit the market at the expense of the poor. The monopsonist would also have other obligations, such as ensuring correct tissue typing to maximize histocompatibility and so minimize graft rejection, and screening for diseased or otherwise hazardous organs and tissues (e.g. HIV infected blood, etc.).

In the United Kingdom, the National Health Service might be ideally suited as our lone purchaser. What we are proposing is that the NHS or a comparable monopsonistic purchaser would purchase live organs and tissues just as it does other goods, for example kidney dialysis machines. It would then make them available as needed at no cost to the recipient.

PRICING POLICY

There may be a problem with pricing policy. In effect, the monopsonist is responsible for the running of the scheme. Should it also be permitted to set the prices of various organs and tissues which it is interested in purchasing? Leaving the pricing of organs to the judgement of the purchaser within a particular marketplace introduces the possibility of a conflict of interests. If the NHS, say, was not only to act as purchaser, but also held responsibility for setting the price of what it purchases, it is not unlikely that it would attempt to set prices as low as possible so as to conserve its resources. However, this would be counterbalanced by the need to provide sufficient incentives to attract would-be organ vendors.

This latter point may provide an option to a mechanism of rigid or fixed prices. It might be thought that in a monopsonistic market there is no possibility for a free market pricing mechanism. However, it must not be forgotten that the monopsonist is under pressure to purchase, this pressure resulting from the need for organs. If the purchaser is responsible for supplying patients with organs, and if there is a demand from the public for such provision, the purchaser will have an obligation to provide organs and a powerful motive for discharging the obligation. This affords the would-be vendor a degree of bargaining power over the price she can demand for her organ. There is an analogy here with the NHS purchasing drugs and other equipment in the current system: in the United Kingdom, even prior to the growth of private sector health care, the position of the NHS as the lone/major purchaser of pharmaceuticals did not afford it the power to dictate the prices of the drugs it purchased.

JUSTICE AND PRIORITY ALLOCATION

It seems to us only right that those who contribute to the scheme and run the risks involved in organ supply, however small they may be, should also be in a position to benefit from the scheme if they one day require an organ – justice demands this much. We would go so far as to say that those who sell their organs and tissues into the marketplace should be afforded greater priority in the allocation of organs if they become patients in need of organs than those who do not, and the responsibility for ensuring priority allocation should lie with the system.

CONFINING THE MARKETPLACE

Wherever payment for organs occurs in the world, whether legally or illegally within a certain jurisdiction, there is a common problem that represents an undesirable effect of the market. It does not seem to be an over-generalization to say that usually the organ vendors come from 'underdeveloped' or 'developing' nations and that, while those who purchase organs may be the 'wealthy' within those nations, because of the disparity in wealth between these and the 'developed' nations (and because, as a general rule, where they exists laws against commerce in organs are less strictly enforced in these nations than in the developed nations), organ purchasers tend more often to be from the latter. Thus it is not surprising that in the recent 'Turkish kidneys for sale' scandal in the United Kingdom, the kidneys removed from the four Turks for payment were used for transplantation in patients at a private hospital in the United Kingdom.[5] In that case, Mr Roger Henderson QC, counsel for the General Medical Council, was reported as saying that '[t]here were great differences in wealth, health and understanding between rich and poor countries which created circumstances in which the rich could prey on the poor unless steps were taken to prevent it'.[6]

One way of preventing rich nations preying on poor ones would be to confine the marketplace, perhaps to a particular nation state, but just as reasonably to a regional bloc of states. We could thus imagine various marketplaces facilitating commerce in live organs and tissues whilst restricting such commerce to the member states of a customs union, or a common market. Several such blocs which might lend themselves readily to our purpose already exist: in Europe, the EU (European Union); in South America, LAFTA (Latin American Free Trade Area), CACM (Central American Common Market), and ACMC (Andean Common Market and Community); in the Caribbean, CARI-COM (Caribbean Economic Community); in Africa, UDEAC (Union Douanière et Economique de l'Afrique Centrale), EAC (East African Community), CEAO (Communauté Economique de l'Afrique de l'Ouest), and ECOWAS (Economic Community of West African States); and in South East Asia, ASEAN (Association of South East Asian Nations).[7] To prevent conflicts of interest, the monopsonist in any one bloc should not be an institution of any particular member state of that bloc, and thus the NHS would be ruled out as the EC's monopsonist, for example.

Confining the marketplace also gets over the problem of organ vendors, or their families not being eligible as organ recipients because they do not reside in the catchment area of a health service managed by the relevant monopsonist. There may be a further reason for confining the marketplace, which is perhaps not very charitable, but one which operates at a practical level and has some rough justice associated with it. We mention it here for what it is worth. It was reported in September 1990 that of 130 patients from the United Arab Emirates and Oman who had purchased kidneys for transplantation from living unrelated 'donors' in Bombay, India, 24 had died within one year of transplantation (Salahudeen *et al.* 1990). Various reasons for this unusually high mortality rate can be postulated, including poor conditions and facilities in Bombay, and the condition of blood products and the purchased kidneys themselves. Three of the patients became seropositive for hepatitis-B during follow up in their home countries, and four were found to be HIV seropositive having tested negative for HIV antibody prior to transplantation. Whilst all blood is routinely tested for HIV in Oman and the UAE, only 5 per cent is checked in Bombay. Thus confining the marketplace would not only prevent depredation of poor states by richer ones, but could also ensure that anyone who has sold her healthy organ into the scheme can expect the same standard of service as the person who received her organ should she later come to need a transplant herself. It seems equitable that organ recipients (or vendors for that matter) of similar age and health within the same marketplace should not face different levels of risk for the same operation.

HUMAN ORGANS *IN VIVO* AS CAPITAL

Consider one particular worry concerning commerce in human biological materials which has been voiced by Andrews (1986 p. 32): 'Allowing payment to living persons for solid organs could lead society to view the poor as suddenly having capital and consequently being ineligible for welfare payments.' We have ruled out compulsory removal of organs from the living, even where the life of another might be at stake – society would find it hard to demand that an individual go under the knife,[8] and such an extreme course would entail so many problems that it would be unlikely to increase the availability of donor organs overall. It is, moreover, unjust for an individual's body parts to be viewed as capital while they remain part of her body. A thinly veiled demand for the individual to realize her capital assets before being eligible for welfare would surely constitute coercion. It is worth emphasizing that nothing we have said rules out altruistic donation as a mode of organ procurement alongside a commercial scheme – we would not wish to discourage donation. However, viewing organs *in vivo* as capital would do just this. If the individual chooses to *donate*, rather than *sell* her kidney, it would be unjust for that individual to be penalized for doing so.

The situation changes only when the individual avails herself of the option to sell her organs. Depending on the price she has been paid for her organ, she might then be liable to a loss of welfare benefits and also to tax. While we note this as a possibility, our suggestion at both a practical and ethical level would be to exempt the profits from organ and tissue sale from tax and also from benefit reduction – an added incentive to sell and a recognition of the residual altruism involved. It should be recognized that when a person sells an organ she acts both selfishly, in advantaging herself, and altruistically, in providing a public service. It might be instructive to compare our attitude to remuneration in the so-called 'caring professions'.

ORGANS, TISSUES AND CELLS USED FOR RESEARCH

Developments in biotechnology rely in no small part on research using human biological materials and thus on their continued availability. Live human derived tissues and cells are used in three main areas of biological research: tissue and cell culture; hybridoma technology; and recombinant DNA technology or genetic engineering (Congress of the United States 1987 Chapter 3). Human tissues and cells may be used in the development of cell lines, hybridomas, and cloned genes, for example, all powerful tools to research scientists. Ultimately, their use may lead to important developments in the diagnostic and therapeutic fields, as well as extending the frontiers of knowledge in the biological sciences.

We have seen that a major moral justification for offering financial incentives to would-be organ vendors in the therapeutic setting is our concern for the vulnerability of those who will die prematurely for the need of an organ transplant. The problem that must be faced in the cases which are our concern here is that no comparable justification seems to exist for asking persons to provide tissues or cells for non-therapeutic research. The question we must ask is: if the reason for asking individuals to provide tissue samples is that their research use will lead to the enlargement of the world scientific knowledge base, or that it might contribute to therapeutic advances, why should they not be paid for those samples?

The particularly hard cases which must be considered in this context are those in which human tissues and cells are required to perform speculative research which, at the outset, it is impossible to predict will lead to anything more than a negative result. Whilst negative results may be useful to scientists – if only to indicate blind alleys to be avoided – these are hard cases ethically because one cannot say categorically, in advance of research being performed, whether the human tissues or cells will be used in the development of anything of benefit to individuals or humankind generally (for example new treatments for disease).

We should set the problem in context. The great majority of living human sources of tissue and cell samples for research purposes are patients. That is, the samples are 'leftovers' (Congress of the United States 1987 p. 51) from biological materials removed for diagnostic purposes or as part of a patient's therapy. Where this is not the case and the source is a research subject, tissue retrieval is usually of minimal risk. Generally, the techniques used involve nothing more than the drawing of a blood sample, or the collection of excretions or secretions (Congress of the United States 1987 p. 51).

PATIENTS

Consider the following scenario. A patient requires a splenectomy as part of her therapy for hairy cell leukaemia (HCL). Research on cells of the patient's removed spleen show her disease to be a very rare T-cell variant of HCL, and scientists establish a productive cell line from the spleen tissue.

This is precisely what happened in the Moore case and is the least morally problematic type of case we have to address here. If the patient's tissue is removed as part of her therapy, then she has not been required to undergo any added risk for the acquisition of a tissue sample than that involved in her therapy. Once the organ has been removed, the mode of disposal of its constituent tissues and cells does not alter the moral terrain.

However let us say that the nature of the patient's disease indicates with certainty that research using the excised tissue will lead to a therapeutic breakthrough which will result in the saving of lives or the alleviation of misery. Where a clear social benefit lies in the research use of her tissue, one may argue from general utility that the patient be denied the option to refuse to transfer title to her tissue. It is not as if the patient is being asked to run any added risk as the tissue has already been removed as part of her therapy. This does not rule out her selling the tissue, but under these conditions the situation is one of compulsory purchase. The patient's original ownership of the tissue is conceded and she is thus entitled to compensation for this mandatory appropriation.

The situation appears to be different where one cannot predict with any certainty that research use of the patient's tissues/cells will lead to anything of general benefit. It may seem wasteful to incinerate the tissue when it could be used for speculative research, but the patient's wishes in the matter should be respected – unless the tissue represents a biohazard, she should be free to take it home, in a brown paper bag if that is what she wants to do. The mere fact that tissues/cells may prove to be of interest to a research scientist does not seem to be a strong enough ground for vitiating a patient's autonomy, or violating her property rights. On the other hand, she may still by her choice donate or sell the tissue. In such cases as these, the patient is in a position to sell her tissue to interested researchers. However, the situation differs from the sale of an organ earmarked for transplantation in that the tissue itself has no direct value, but acquires its value from its use in the research process. Thus a sale at the point of treatment system would not be a particularly efficient solution at a practical level. For one thing, most patients, it is fair to assume, would not be in a position to know the true value of, and consequently what price to ask for their excised tissues. We could introduce into the system some mechanism for the valuation prior to sale of tissues removed at surgery, but those best suited to perform valuations are likely to be research scientists and thus it would be difficult to avoid conflicts of interests.

A better system would be one where the patient is afforded a percentage share of any profits which come of the research use of her tissues or cells. The need for valuation of tissues/cells at the point of treatment is then obviated since, much as with a royalty system, the patient's profits are determined by the sales of any product(s) derived from her tissues. But how are we to decide what percentage of those profits is to be assigned to the patient? The problem is that, as in the Moore case, the tissue may be used in the derivation of a cell line or some other research tool, and it is this, not the tissue itself, that is of commercial value. Notwithstanding our having taken as a starting premise that the patient owns her excised tissue, a cell line is not a product of the human body (Erin 1994). The source tissue is crucial to the derivation of a cell line, and this is what affords the patient bargaining power, but it is only one of several factors involved in the line's creation. The problem is exacerbated if it is not the cell line that is valuable, in pecuniary terms, but some product in the development of which the line has played a part. Should the patient be assigned a share in profits which may accrue from a secondary derivative of her tissues, that is, a product developed using a cell line derived from her cells? Moreover, where biomedical research use of human tissues and cells does result in a profitable product, it is often the case that biological materials from many human sources have been involved in the process.

RESEARCH SUBJECTS

Unlike the procurement of tissues and cells from patients, in procurement from research subjects the removal of tissues and cells is not intended to benefit, therapeutically, the individual who is their source. Ethically, this is similar to organ retrieval from the living already discussed. Where there is a significant moral difference it is in the need for tissues and the purpose to which they are to be put. Unlike organs for transplantation, there is no direct beneficiary of tissues and cells destined for research use. However, if excised tissues and cells were to contribute, albeit in the long term, to the development of, say, a cure for cancer, this would be seen as a major benefit to humankind and the cure would certainly save lives. No case can be made for the compulsory removal from a living person of tissue/cell samples for research use,[9] but if the individual makes an autonomous decision to supply samples for a cancer research protocol, for example, there is no moral reason why she should not be paid for the sample rather than donate it.

The hard cases are, again, those in which it cannot be predicted whether research use of excised tissues and cells will, eventually, lead to a therapeutic advance. Research use may lead to a therapeutic advance, but is this a sufficient justification for providing financial incentives in tissue/cell procurement? We would say that where the human tissue samples are needed for speculative research, as long as the research subject is not required to undergo more than a minimal risk of harm in supplying a sample and is not coerced into doing so, there is no moral reason why she should not sell her property.

AN OPEN MARKET?

When discussing the procurement of human organs for therapeutic purposes, our main concern was to devise a commercial scheme which would make up the shortfall in donated organs for transplantation. In the context of human tissues and cells needed for biomedical research purposes, our aim should be to maximize the potential of that research to yield therapeutic advances whilst safeguarding the autonomy of the individual who is the source of tissues/cells (and so preventing her exploitation) and respecting her property rights. To prevent richer nations preying on poorer ones in the former case, we proposed confining the marketplace. However, this does not seem appropriate in the research setting. The legal protection of property rights by the granting of patents is a well established practice, and temporary secrecy to protect ongoing research is tolerated and may in fact be desirable (Bok 1986 p. 160), but, in the academic environment at least, openness and the rapid publishing of results in refereed journals are chief elements of the scientific ethos.[10] Worldwide dissemination of research results enhances the capacity for research to lead to useful developments in therapeutics. Furthermore, even where a research tool such as a cell line has been patented, the patentee will often provide samples to other interested researchers: indeed, in the Moore affair, Professor Golde made samples of the Mo cell line available to other scientific establishments *gratis* (Golde 1984).

It seems likely that confining research use of human tissues to the marketplace in which they were purchased may be an obstacle to maximizing the tissues' full research potential. We therefore propose that the monopsonist within a particular marketplace be free to sell, or license the use of, or supply *gratis* tissue samples to monopsonists in other marketplaces. Any profits which may be yielded by doing so would be distributed throughout the system.

TAX REBATES

It should be apparent from the foregoing discussion that the practical problems presented by an attempt to commercialize the procurement of human biological materials for research purposes are greater and more complex than in the case of organs needed for therapy. Firstly, there is the question of whether patients or research subjects should profit from second or third order products, that is, for example, whether they should profit from a product developed using a tool derived from the tissues they supply. If we were to introduce a percentage share system, should the individual's right to share in profits last in perpetuity? Should it be transferable to her heirs? If we accept that where an individual's tissues have been used in the development of a profitable product she should share in those profits, should we not also require that the individual share in the costs of research where no profitable product is developed? And so on.

One possible scheme which would circumvent these practical difficulties and at the same time concede the property issue and emphasize the public interest in the research use of human biological materials is a system whereby incentives in the form of discounts against tax are provided for the supply of human tissues/cells for research. Research subjects would have ultimate control over the disposition of their *in vivo* tissues, but where research scientists wish to use those tissues and the research subject consents to removal for research use and transfers title to them to the monopsonist, she receives consideration in the form of tax relief. The patient whose 'leftovers' are used for research would also be afforded tax relief.

One reason we suggest a tax rebate system, as opposed to a lump sum cash system as in the organs for therapy situation, is that such a system sends out the right messages. Firstly, any tax system recognizes that what a citizen pays in tax is originally owned by that citizen,[11] and the individual's ownership of her tissues is thus ratified. Secondly, the research use of human tissues is ultimately intended to serve the commonweal. There is a general interest in the procurement of a tissue sample – this may lie in the enhancement of the scientific knowledge base, or in therapeutic advances – as opposed to the direct benefit to the individual which the procurement of an organ provides. And this is a chief foundation of modern day tax systems: funds raised through the levying of taxes on individuals are used for the benefit of all citizens in the provision of public services. Thus the offering of a discount against tax for supplying of tissue samples for research use may also be viewed as a premium for the provision of a public service.

Though the rich may pay more in taxes, they are not eligible for preferential treatment in the use of public services. Even if an individual's tissues were used in the development of a highly profitable product, the profits made by the monopsonist would be distributed throughout the system and for the equitable benefit of all who are subject to it, and would not return to the individual in any greater degree than to any other citizen.

What of the poverty stricken citizen who pays little in tax, or the individual who is eligible for state welfare benefits? It is true that in nations such as the United Kingdom all citizens are subject to Value Added Tax, but offering rebates against VAT would likely prove so complicated as to be impracticable. It might be thought that a system offering rewards in the form of discounts on tax would mean little or nothing to the poorer members of society. However, we see no reason why those whose tax burden is less than the value of the tax discounts received for tissues supplied should not be offered tax refunds, just as is the person who overpays her income tax.

Whilst we believe a tax discount system would adequately deal with many of the problems presented by the commercialization of tissue procurement for research use, various difficulties remain. For example, at what level should tax relief be set? Should that level be standardized for types of tissues, or should it vary – $\alpha\%$ for blood, $\beta\%$ for plasma, $\gamma\%$ for tumour material, etc? Should tax credits be redeemable for one tax year? Two? Several? Furthermore, we should not forget that we are discussing marketplaces comprising separate nation states, and it is not necessarily the case that member states within a bloc have similar tax systems or, where they do not, that they would submit readily to a common taxation policy. The monopsonist would thus need to negotiate with each state in the bloc within which it functions.

RESTATEMENT OF RATIONALE

Our purpose in this chapter has been principally to recommend the ethics of a monopsonistic market for organs and tissues. We have here been less concerned with the ethics of the marketplace *per se* than with working out how at least one sort of market might function ethically. We should emphasize that the underlying justification for a monopsonistic market in human organs and tissues is not a concomitant to the ethic of the free market, but is a response to the moral pressure created by the needs of those who require human organs and tissues either to preserve their very lives or in order to carry out research in the public interest.

NOTES

1. *Moore v The Regents of the University of California*, Case No.C513755 (September ll, 1984, Cal. Super. Ct LA). Though John Moore filed suit in 1984, the decision of the Supreme Court of California was not handed down until July 9, 1990. For a review of the case see, for example, Freeman (1994) or Erin (1994).
2. One could imagine reasons why a living person would wish to sell a vital organ – to benefit loved ones for example. Whether this is morally objectionable depends on whether it is morally legitimate to sacrifice one's own life to save that of another.
3. As is argued in the context of blood supply by Titmuss (1972). For an response to Titmuss, see, for example, Arrow (1972).
4. Lori B. Andrews (1986 p. 32) makes a similar point: 'Society has not benefited individuals by banning organ sales unless it also provides a means to escape desperate conditions.'
5. For press coverage of the affair see *The Times* (London),December 4, 5, 7, 8, 9, 13, 14 and 15, 1989; January 10, 11, 18, 19, 20 and 25, 1990; February 17, 21, 22, 24, 27 and 28, 1990; March 27, 28, 29, 30 and 31, 1990; April 3 and 5, 1990.
6. As reported in *The Times* (London), December 5, 1989, p. 1.
7. For the respective member states of these blocs see Dicken (1986 p. 146).

8. See Harris (1975), but remember that here we are dealing with what would be attractive and effective at a practical level.
9. There are cases in which the State can legally demand a tissue sample (for example, in the United Kingdom a blood or urine sample can be demanded under the Road Traffic Act 1972), but this is not one of them.
10. In the current climate of widespread commercialization of biotechnology, R. K. Merton's characterization of the ethos of science (1942) has become outmoded and now appears idealistic, but his 'communism' remains a scientific imperative.
11. This remains true even where the citizen is taxed at source and the money paid in tax never comes into her hands – though she may not have the freedom to dispose of it, the money is recognized as owned by her originally.

REFERENCES

Andrews, L. B. (1986), 'My body, my property', *Hastings Center Report*, XVI, pp. 28–38
Arrow, K. J. (1972), 'Gifts and exchanges', *Philosophy and Public Affairs*, I, pp. 343–62
Bok, S. (1986), *Secrets: On The Ethics of Concealment and Revelation*, Oxford University Press
Brams, M. (1977), 'Transplantable human organs: should their sale be authorized by state statutes?', *American Journal of Law and Medicine*, III, pp. 183–95
Buc, N. L. and Bernstein, J. Z. (1984), 'Buying and selling human organs is worth a harder look', *Health-Scan*, I, pp. 3–5
Congress of the United States, Office of Technology Assessment (1987), *New Developments In Biotechnology: Ownership Of Human Tissues And Cells*, Special Report OTA-BA–337, US Government Printing Office, Washington, DC
Dicken, P. (1986), *Global Shift: Institutional Change In a Turbulent World*, Harper and Row, London
Erin, C. A. (1994) 'Who owns Mo?: Using historical entitlement theory to decide the ownership of human derived cell lines', in A. O. Dyson and J. Harris (eds), *Ethics and Biotechnology*, Routledge, London, 157–78
Erin, C. A. and Harris, J. (1991), 'Surrogacy' *Bailliere's Clinical Obstetrics, and Gynaecology*, 5th edition, pp. 611–35
Freeman, M. D. A. (1994), 'Biotechnology, patients and profits: how is the law to respond?' (Chapter 8 this volume)
Golde, D. W. (1984), 'Availability of Mo and HTLV-II', *Nature*, CCCVIII, p. 19
Harris, J. (1975), 'The survival lottery', *Philosophy*, L, pp. 81–7
—— (1991), 'Commercial exploitation', a revised and contracted version of Harris 1992 (Chapters 5 and 6), presented at the Manchester Political Theory Conference, Children: Their Rights; Our Obligations, Department of Government, University of Manchester, November 29, 1991
—— (1992), *Wonderwoman And Superman: The Ethics Of Human Biotechnology*, Oxford University Press
Honore, A. M. (1961), 'Ownership', in A. G. Guest, (ed.), *Oxford Essays In Jurisprudence*, Oxford University Press, 107–47
Merton, R. K. (1942), 'Science and technology in a democratic order', *Journal of Legal And Political Sociology*, I
Munzer, S. R. (1990), *A Theory of Property*, Cambridge University Press
Salahudeen, A. K., Woods, H. F., Pingle, A., Nur-EI-Huda Suleyman, M., Shakuntala,

K., Nandakumar, M., Yahya, T. M., and Daar, A. S. (1990), 'High mortality among recipients of bought living-unrelated donor kidneys', *Lancet*, CCCXXXVI, pp. 725–8

Scowen, E. (1990), 'The human body: whose property and whose profit?', *Discovery*, I, pp. 1–3

Schwarz, C., Davidson, G., Seaton, A., and Tebbit, V. (eds.), (1988), *Chambers English Dictionary*, W. and R. Chambers, Cambridge

Titmuss, R. (1972), *The Gift Relationship: From Human Blood To Social Policy*, Pantheon, New York

Warnock, M. (1985), *A Question Of Life: The Warnock Report On Human Fertilization and Embryology*, Basil Blackwell, Oxford

PART THREE

The cultural context of choice in relation to high technology medicine

10

How can good choices be made about dying?

ROGER HIGGS

Choice in medicine, as well as in relation to high technology, can be seen to be loosely but quite clearly connected. When Mozart lay dying 200 years ago, we know of few options open to him. Whatever condition he was dying from, which could not be accurately diagnosed, there was no question of rational treatment. Without potentially active treatment, no elective medical choices could be made in terms which would be currently understood.

Therefore it may seem that real choices in medicine have only appeared historically with the emergence of modern medicine. That is first with the development of accurate diagnosis but, in effect, only with the arrival of treatment options which can affect outcome. Such treatments themselves have largely occurred as the result of scientific and technical advances. These advances have been so rapid that succeeding generations have needed to fix the boundaries between ordinary medical responses, and extraordinary high technology medicine so that they each occur in totally different places.

Yet, however simple the 'white pills' that people swallow may look, their abilities to kill bacteria or alter the function of the kidneys are the product of sophisticated and refined technological advances. Thus, choice, medicine and high technology are inextricably connected. Although it may be clearer now what is considered as 'high technology', the concept is a dynamic and a changing one. As a general practitioner, I am therefore interested in the effects which the growing technological edge of modern medicine has had, and will have on our society, and I want to examine in particular its effects on choices that are made about dying. However before examining this issue it is important to consider the general context in which such debates are taking place.

The focus of this exploration therefore will be partly on values in relation to medical practice. The importance now given to a consideration of values is at least one clear consequence of the explosion in high technology. Ethical discussions at medical schools (Pond 1987), or in medical staff rooms is now not unusual, and indeed much of the debate in this collection is based on the assumption that an open and explicit approach to ethical issues is important. Fifty years ago I am assured that such a situation did not exist. Certainly when I was a medical student in the 1960s, medical ethics was still considered a fringe and rather suspect activity. Such teaching as there was in this area was mostly concerned with professional activities and boundaries, and could be characterised as based on a 'trade union' view of medical ethics. The stimulus which has brought ethical considerations near to the centre stage has been the emergence of new, high technology treatments which have changed categories and created dilemmas of choice – for example in the challenge of deciding what to do with severely malformed neonates, or to whom to give kidney transplants. These kinds of challenges are those largely for physicians and health planners to debate, and although they are a legitimate part of this discussion, I largely disregard them for I wish to concentrate on those choices available to the majority of people who will die at older ages in different circumstances. However it is important to acknowledge in passing that these dilemmas have spawned the most vigorous current debate – that is, how to allocate the clearly finite resources which can be devoted to health care even in the richest countries of our small planet.

Nonetheless the focus of my examination is on choices, not for those professionally concerned with health care but for people at large, particularly patients, who find themselves making such choices in the context of high technology medicine when facing a terminal illness. It is in this area of ordinary, day-to-day ethics – which focuses on what people should say to each other in such situations, and on what role people should have in making choices and decisions – which has always been my interest (Campbell and Higgs 1982). Whilst this debate has existed as long as there has been medical care of those with terminal illness, it was never considered as a legitimate area for general discussion, nor indeed was seen as a legitimate area for philosophers, sociologists and theoretical lawyers to consider – that is, before medical ethics emerged from the shadows with the advent of high technology medicine.

Another effect of high technology medicine has been to invest its purveyors with a special status, which generally I should not like to challenge. However, the effects on ordinary health care have been less than satisfactory. Fifty years ago the status of the ordinary doctor could not have been lower. In the intervening period there has been a tendency for both patients and practitioners to assume that a specialist, who knows a lot about a little, is now an even more powerful figure than the generalist, who knows a little about a lot. Although the debate about the relative roles of generalists and specialists has been sterile, it runs through the provision of health care. Some ill people are very attracted to centres of high technology, and may be caused personal harm – in addition to that caused to health care budgets – if they are treated in a high technology style when they have a low technology illness. An example might be a brain scan for a tension headache (Dale *et al.* 1991).

This issue raises questions which might not emerge elsewhere about the assumptions underlying our general choices between high and low technology. The problem may be best asked in the form of the following question: why should we choose the 'lowest-possible tech' solution to a problem in health care, when such an approach is not used, for example, in broadcasting or in transportation (*pace* Illich 1975)? All things being otherwise equal, the answer may be based on a range of factors. One such factor undoubtedly relates to the elegance of the technology – a simple solution always seems to be preferred. Such a solution would appeal to a latter-day William of Occam saying that 'Entities are not to be multiplied beyond necessity' (Russell 1946). Another reason for advocating or supporting low technology solutions might be that of parsimony and good housekeeping. Low technology solutions probably mean lower cost, which is likely to be associated at the same time with being more environmentally friendly or 'greener'. In addition to using less un-renewable resources such solutions may also have the virtue of lessening the gap between those who are rich and those who are poor.

There are in addition substantial commercial imperatives in high technology development. For example, the pressure on pharmaceutical and other companies producing medical products to recoup development costs by obtaining large and increasing sales, and by disguising sales activity as research. In this respect Preston, Chapter 7, discusses one such example of the considerable commercial pressures attached to the development of the artificial heart. Such pressures create an effect on all prescribers and patients. Everyone wishes to obtain the latest and most technologically sophisticated product.

But perhaps the most potent point of discussion about the bases upon which choices are made at the time of dying is whether high technology interventions have a depersonalising effect on their users. In my experience there is a nightmare in many people's minds that they may die, surrounded by tubes, bottles, pumps and machines, without personal warmth and comfort. As one commentator recently described a woman in intensive care. 'For several weeks she was known simply as "Bed No. 3" '(Evans 1991). The perception of such a nightmare may be unfair in view of the clear achievements of high technology medicine. Moreover, usually the criticism relates to the ways in such medicine is used, and is not directed at its basic function. Nonetheless, the dilemma that is posed by excessive and unthinking use of high technology medicine does need to be recognised when the choices that people make, or might like to make when they are faced with a lethal prognosis, are examined. Now that life expectancy has considerably increased in many advanced industrialised countries – itself a change assisted in part by effective medical care – people need to fear dying prematurely less and less. However their fears now focus far more on the mode of death.

In considering the mode and timing of death it is worth reflecting on the meaning of the word 'euthanasia' which can be understood as basically and simply 'a good death', and further investigating what such a good death might now be thought to be. In practice one of the most important issues to be considered in relation to the process of dying must be the control of physical symptoms such as pain, vomiting and diarrhoea. If such symptoms are stabilised or checked, bodily processes become less chaotic, and are perceived to be more under the persons's control. In addition the control of what might be called 'mental' symptoms – the potential chaos of the mind at such a time – through the reduction of the effects of such things as depression, panic and sleeplessness, is particularly important.

However, this vision of control of both symptoms of the body and mind is now challenged by an understanding that sadness is inevitably part of dying. The denial of the inevitability of sadness by treating, or what might be called 'high teching' it out of the way, makes many of those professionally concerned with people at such a time feel uneasy. Although at the point of death many people may appear socially withdrawn, either because of the mental clouding which may occur at such a time, or through drawing back into their own worlds, our image of the good death must now begin to include companionship. Essentially such companionship must mean choosing who those people are with whom one wants to be at that time. The idea of companionship must additionally include both personal and physical contact, and self respect and dignity which is set in the framework of special personal relationships.

It may be the case that the loneliness of old age is beyond all technological aid. In very old age, for example at the age of 90, very few friends are still likely to be alive, and the fear of dying in such circumstances is hard to banish. Nevertheless even in this situation, pride in, and understanding the meaning of what is past, and making sense of what this particular person and their individual life has meant, creates an intensely significant experience for them. The experience is expressed in the need to continue to be oneself and somehow, by being in control and by looking and feeling one's best, to be able still to make some choices.

Thus, although high technology approaches show promise, at least for controlling certain symptoms and for palliation, there has been a recent realisation that they may inhibit personal and professional responses to individuals' emotional needs. Such problems either may occur early in the final illness, when crucial decisions about the type of care or direction of treatment are made, or they may occur in the final days. At this latter point a peaceful death may be denied to the person concerned, because the disease, and the persistent struggle against it continues to be the focus of the medical care provided (Cohen 1993).

To illustrate some of the points in the commentary above about making good choices at the time of dying, I now include a discussion of four real case histories, published in the *Journal of Medical Ethics*, which seem to reflect particularly important issues which must be considered in the medical care of people at this time of their lives.

In 'a case of obstructed death' (Higgs 1982) the case history of a woman is presented who, after a chest operation which revealed inoperable cancer, was lied to about her diagnosis. As a result she lived her final moments in 'limbo' as it were, without the possibility of open communication with her spouse, or her doctors. This sort of story presented in all its starkness must be less common now: few could defend the giving of false information in such a way. However, the intention to preserve hope by all means remains a difficulty for professional and personal carers in terminal illness. Truth telling is a complex area I have studied elsewhere (Higgs 1985), but the conclusions are clear. Although there will be some who do not wish to enter into discussion about their future, and they must be handled sensitively, the majority of people appear to want, and undoubtedly deserve, clear information about issues of such importance to them. Nonetheless clear information may he difficult to give when the patient is desperately ill, or when the procedures used are high technology ones: such procedures may be extremely complex to administer, or they have many possible outcomes, or in some sense they may still be experimental and under development (see Chapter 6). In the case of experimental procedures they may be covered by regulations, or be improved by scrutiny from an ethics committee. However this does not exempt professional carers from providing information on the basis of which individual patients can make their own choices, however emotionally difficult these choices may be.

Recourse to legal clarification of what is meant in practice by informed consent has been of some help in many countries recently. However undue reliance on the legal basis of informed consent has led some centres to produce written information of such quantity and complexity that it is, in effect, only comprehensible as a basis on which to make choices by those who are highly intelligent, motivated and completely well. Whilst there has been a good response to the challenge of medical truthfulness in relation to diagnosis, outcomes and treatment in the fields of cancer and AIDS – often assisted by the prompting of voluntary organisations in Britain such as BACUP for those with cancer and various AIDS charities – the general level of understanding amongst those with terminal conditions is still variable, and the skills of the professionals concerned with giving information correspondingly still underdeveloped.

With the breadth of the field so wide, and change so rapid, information giving at a point of clinical crisis remains an area of major concern. Trust between the patient and those caring for them is a delicate issue, and such trust may be the only effective 'therapy' in some conditions both currently, and for the foreseeable future. Even if treatments do become available, their efficacy is likely to be lessened if mutual understanding is poor, or mistrust is pronounced in the doctor-patient relationship. Therefore, paradoxically, it may be that decisions over the use of high technology procedures in terminal care have shown how much good social and personal relationships are needed.

It may still be the case that even when options are explained and are available, that the person who is dying may still wish to take the road least favoured by medical and nursing attendants. In 'earning his morphine' (Higgs *et al.* 1987) the case is presented of an elderly

feeding, or the implanted venous injection sites so much used in the care of patients with AIDS are examples of technological developments in everyday use. The knowledge that this kind of technology is acceptable and accessible – and not impersonal, cold or alien – is of enormous relief to people, and enables them to take control of their lives in their own environment. These developments enable people to maintain their usual relationships and activities often until the very end. These relationships, too, are strengthened by the process of sharing in the care. Helpers and relatives who can now do things that previously only nurses used to do may find openness created between them as high technology medicine is brought down to, and understood and used on a human scale.

From this final discussion we can discern another important aim for high technology medicine in relation to the management of a good death – that it should help to enhance relationships between people at such an important time. Joint ownership of the situation, and shared decisions about it can lead to the healing of relationships when there is no final bodily healing possible for one of the parties. The proper and extended handling of the shock of a terminal diagnosis, which Kfir and Slevin (1991) describe as a form of crisis intervention, is precisely the response that we need to consider in relation to a high technology intervention. With this sort of model, proper care can be set up not only for the patient, but for relatives and for professional carers. A good death sets up the possibility of the reasonable bereavement, and with that perhaps the chance of better choices for the future of our society at large.

REFERENCES

British Medical Association, (1988), *Working Party to Review the BMA's Guidelines on Euthanasia: the Euthanasia Report*, BMA, London

Campbell, A. and Higgs, R. (1982), *In That Case: Medical Ethics in Everyday Practice*, Darton, Longman and Todd, London

Cohen, S. (1993), *Whose Life is it Anyhow?*, Robson Books, London

Dale, J., Green, J., Glucksman, E., and Higgs, R. (1991), *Providing for Primary Care: Progress in A and E*, London

Evans, D. (1991), Paper presented to Society of Anaesthetists

Higgs, R. (1982), 'Truth at the last: a case of obstructed death?', *Journal of Medical Ethics*, x, pp. 48–50

—— (1983), 'Cutting the thread and pulling the wool: a request for euthanasia in general practice', *Journal of Medical Ethics*, ix, pp. 45–9

—— (1984), 'Kicking against the pricks: two patients wish to end essential insulin treatment', *Journal of Medical Ethics*, x, pp. 201–8

—— (1985), 'On telling patients the truth', in Lockwood M. (ed.), *Dilemmas in Modern Medicine*, Oxford University Press

—— (1987), 'Living wills and treatment refusal', *British Medical Journal*, CCLXLV, pp. 1221–2

—— (1988), 'Not the last word on euthanasia', *British Medical Journal*, CCLXLVI, p. 1348

Higgs, R., Livesley, B., Rennie, J., and relatives. (1987), 'Earning his heroin but seeking release while the surgeon advises amputation', *Journal of Medical Ethics*, XIII, pp. 43–8

Illich, I. (1975), *Medical Nemesis*, Calder and Boyars, London

Institute of Medical Ethics Working Party (1990), 'Assisted death', *Lancet*, CCCXXXVI, pp. 610–13

Kfir, N. and Slevin. M. (1991), 'Crisis intervention with cancer patients', in R. Comey (ed.), *Developing Counselling and Communication Skills in Medicine*, Routledge, London

Pond, D. (1987), *Report of a Working Party on the Teaching of Medical Ethics*, Institute of Medical Ethics Publications, London

Russell, B. (1946), *History of Western Philosophy*, George Allen and Unwin, London, p. 462

11

Contests with death: ideologies of nationalism and internationalism in Japan

MARGARET LOCK

In North America and to a lesser extent in Europe, at the core of the current rhetoric on bioethics, stands the concept of individual rights. In the abortion debate, for example, the most public and contentious of disputes, anti-abortion advocates build their argument around the rights of the foetus, while pro-choice advocates focus on the rights of the mother, and assign the foetus to a pre-juridical status. But if we look beyond what appears to be simply an argument about definitions of non-life and life, it becomes evident that the debate is not merely over the status of abortion, nor is it simply to do with the rights of individuals, but is also about something much more pervasive: gender conflict and the position of women in society today (Faludi: 1991).

The present situation in Japan stands in sharp contrast to that in North America. Japan is a nation where historically the collective imagination has been fascinated with death, where the notion of individual rights is often equated with selfishness, and where no concept of the right to life has ever taken root. For the majority of Japanese, the foetus is simply part of the mother's flesh, and until recently a newborn child was not regarded as fully human for several days after birth. A few Japanese feminists and several representatives of the New Religions raise the question of abortion for discussion (for very different reasons). However, so far this subject has been subject to relatively little public debate despite abortion having been the major form of birth control in Japan until recently. It is now super-seded only by the condom, for the pill is still not legally available for contraceptive purposes. This does not mean, however, that an aborted foetus has no symbolic value its soul can prey on the living, and a lucrative side-line offered by Buddhist temples is the sale of expensive talismans and statues to guilt-ridden women. It is a guilt which must be repeatedly assuaged. Nevertheless, the legality and morality of abortion is not usually contested. Women are relatively matter-of-fact about it, and will report their own experiences with little reservation. At a more general level, the assumption that women, working or otherwise, should have as their prime function in society the nurturing of others, infants, children, husbands, and elderly relatives, is not widely disputed, even though many women are quite well appraised of feminist issues in the West. Hence, although people are saddened and sometimes guilty about the suffering which they may have caused to an unwanted foetus, abortion, despite its potential as a contentious issue, does not function in Japanese society at the present time as a potent signifier for debate about either individual rights or gender roles.

Again in contrast to the West, the question of death has commanded public attention in Japan for more than 20 years and with a growing intensity to such an extent that all other medically related ethical issues have received relatively little attention. The main contested issue relates to the suffering of terminally ill or severely damaged people and whether, when the brain stops functioning, they are in fact still alive. However, perusal of various texts makes it clear that the subjective experience of patients and a concern for their needs in this debate is virtually obliterated in a larger discussion very familiar to analysts of Japan, replete with a rhetoric about contradictions between tradition and modernity, authority and subjectivity, family obligations and individual needs. This is a rhetoric which is very often couched in comparisons, both implicit and explicit, between Self and Other, 'Japan' and the 'West'.

The highly stylized Japanese dramatical form known as Noh has been a forum since the fourteenth century for an exploration of the relationship between the world of spirits and earthly life. The conservative tradition of Noh means it is very rare indeed for written work later than the mid-nineteenth century to enter the consecrated canon and be performed in public. However, in 1991 a play entitled *The Well of Ignorance*, the creation of an eminent Tokyo immunologist, which premiered at the National Noh theatre to a full house, was subsequently scheduled to be repeated on national television.

The play is about a fisherman knocked unconscious in a giant storm, who is taken for dead. The wealthy father of a young woman who is very ill summons a traditional Chinese-style doctor who removes the fisherman's heart and uses it to save the woman's life. The ensuing drama focuses both on the plight of the donor of the heart, who remains hovering in the world of restless spirits, neither alive or dead, and the guilt which racks the young woman for having caused this misery. The narrative in Noh is furnished by a chorus of chanters accompanied by traditional musical instruments, and it is through them that the spirit of the fisherman describes the removal of his own heart.:

> When I was barely hanging on to life, the doctors decided to come at me with blades and scissors. They opened my chest and took my beating heart out and I heard the sounds of snipping and cutting. But my body was totally frozen, and no voice came out when I screamed!
> Am I living, or am I dead?

In characteristic Japanese form, the ambiguity is not resolved by the end of the play, the spirit remains suspended, restless, mutilated, and the young woman's efforts to purify herself at the village well prove fruitless when it dries up, caused, according to the frightened villagers, by a curse. The immunologist playwright Dr Tada claims that he personally has no objection to organ transplants. However, the inertia in the world of Noh which had to be overcome to have the drama produced in public, and the powerful emotional responses he set out to create in the audience belie his words – especially since his play is about the most controversial bioethical issue in Japan today. In choosing the medium of Noh and not the contemporary theatre, Dr Tada was able to give the drama mythological dimensions; to infuse it with mystical and nostalgic associations. The play can be read simply as an allegory for the current national debate in Japan about the acceptability or otherwise of brain death. However at the same time, it is clear that it represents much more than this, particularly because use is made of the tradition of Noh. It is designed expressly to subtly unify the audience by drawing on and rekindling their shared sensitivity to the unique qualities widely attributed to being Japanese.

The fuel for the present discussion about death was ignited in 1968 in Sapporo when Japan's first and only heart transplant to date was carried out by a physician who was subsequently prosecuted on a charge of murder, but eventually acquitted after six years of wrangling. The majority of Japanese people believe today that in that particular case the patient whose heart was removed was not brain dead, and that the recipient, who died two and a half months after the operation, was not sufficiently in need of a new heart to have undergone the transplant. As part of the current national debate discussion about this case was reopened in 1991. The chair of the Japanese Medical Association, when asked to testify before a government committee on brain death and organ transplants, reported that twenty-three years ago, right after the removal of the supposedly ineffective original heart from the recipient, it had been tampered with, thus indicating that the involved doctors may have tried to exaggerate the degree of its deterioration (*Mainichi Shinbun*: 1991a). In short, the case is now generally considered in retrospect as a barbarous piece of medical experimentation carried out by a doctor who, significantly, had received a good portion of his training in America.

There have been other cases in connection with organ transplants where judgements of members of the Japanese medical profession have been seriously challenged. One involved a highly controversial kidney/pancreas transplant at Tsukuba University in which organs were taken from a young mentally retarded woman who was purportedly brain dead. However, neither she nor her parents had given permission for the removal of the organs (*Mainichi Daily News*: 1984). In another instance in 1989 a doctor at the Hamamatsu National Medical School hospital was arrested and charged with swindling more than 20 million yen (about $180,000) from a patient by offering to find a donor for a kidney transplant which the patient needed. The patient died one day after handing the money over, having been told by the doctor that the large fee was necessary for recompense (*sharei*) to the organ donor (*Asahi Shinbun*: 1989). Whilst it is illegal to buy and sell human organs in Japan, there is a long standing custom of giving substantial 'thank you presents' to doctors for special care received. Thus many people believe that commercialization of the organ trade is a realistic possibility, and perhaps in some cases already in operation.

In 1991 a team of physicians appeared in a newspaper photograph defiantly lined up side by side, having decided to go public some months after the actual event about a kidney transplant which they had undertaken using a brain dead donor (*Mainichi Daily News*: 1991a). Although it is not essential to use a brain dead donor for a kidney transplant, physicians judge at times that there is a better chance of successful surgery if the organ is very 'fresh'. Whilst it is estimated that more than 200 kidney transplants have been carried out in Japan from brain dead donors who are usually close relatives of the recipients, details of these procedures are rarely made public.

In a recent case a patient was declared brain-dead by a medical team, and his kidneys were removed for donation. Later it was revealed that although the family had given assent they were not informed at the time that their relative was brain dead and that his heart was still beating. When confronted with the situation one of the surgeons involved stated that, 'it didn't even occur to me to tell the family that I was removing the organs after their relative was pronounced brain-dead; they were eager to donate his kidneys and the chances of success were higher with fresh organs, so I went ahead with it' (*Mainichi Shinbun*: 1991b).

More recently, in full view of the nation as it watched on television, police entered Osaka University Hospital to issue a warning to surgeons that they should not remove the liver of a patient. In this case the 51 year old man had provided in his will that his organs could be made available for transplants, and approval had also been obtained from his family. After being hit by a car the man was taken in an unconscious state to a nearby hospital, and then transferred to Osaka University Hospital with the intention of having his liver and other organs removed after he had been declared brain dead on three occasions by different teams of doctors. The police declared that an autopsy was legally necessary after the car accident. They also reminded doctors that brain death is not legal in Japan, and warned physicians to wait until the heart had stopped beating. Television viewers were treated to the sight of police marching purposively along hospital corridors, whilst defiant doctors shut doors in the face of both television cameras and the police. By the time the liver was eventually removed it had degenerated badly and was unusable. However, the kidneys and pancreas were extracted and transplanted into other patients. This incident triggered revelations that this was not the first case where police had intervened and prevented physicians from removing organs from brain dead donors.

In January 1988, after two years of meetings by a working group, the directors of the Japan Medical Association voted unanimously to accept brain death as the termination of human life. Despite this decision there remains a lack of agreement among the medical profession who are deeply divided on the issue. The Japan Neurologists' Association, for example, in spite of the ruling of the JMA, has rejected brain death as a diagnosis for death. They fear that such a definition will lead to the risk that handicapped, mentally impaired, and disadvantaged patients will be diagnosed prematurely as brain dead in order to remove their organs.

Some physicians have joined members of the public to form the highly visible Patients' Rights Committee, whose interests are not restricted to the question of brain death. Under the leadership of a doctor from the prestigious department of internal medicine at Tokyo University they have recently filed several law suits charging murder when organs have been removed from brain dead patients. One charge was in connection with the Tsukuba University case described above, and another involved a Niigata hospital in which the kidneys of a brain dead patient had been removed. In both these cases the public prosecutor declined to reach a decision. Eventually the cases were thrown out of court, the prosecutor stating as he did so that there was no public consensus in Japan as to how to define death (Nakayama: 1989).

The government has had a series of advisory panels in place since 1983 to consider the question of brain death, culminating in late 1989 in a Special Cabinet Committee on Brain Death and Organ Transplants. This committee, composed of fifteen members from various walks of life, was charged with making a report to the prime minister by 1991. The group was so deeply divided that for a while it appeared that nothing more than an interim report would be produced. However in January 1992 a final report did materialize. The members should have achieved consensus, but they could not do so. The majority position in the report is that brain death is equivalent to human death, that organ transplants from brain dead donors are acceptable, and that the current definition of brain death as formulated by the Ministry of Health is appropriate. A minority position made clear that the social and cultural aspects of the problem should be fully debated, for in this view the debate thus far has been largely confined to inadequate 'scientific' information. Through information publicly available, it is evident that many of those who testified before the committee, including certain scientists and doctors, have argued against acceptance of brain death, but nevertheless the majority of the members eventually moved to support its approval (*Nihon Keizai Shinbun*: 1992). The matter is therefore now back in the hands of the government. Whatever decision is made – if one is formally made at all – it is unlikely to incite a flood of organ transplantations because of the probable shortage of donors.

In the meantime the Japan Federation of Bar Associations

(Nichibenren) has made a public statement to the effect that brain death should not be accepted as the point at which life is terminated. In its report a concern was expressed for the 'sanctity of life', and about the consequences for possible medical 'experimentation.' The Federation also pointed out the lack of public consensus of the issue and that there may be unforeseen consequences in connection with inheritance claims (*Mainichi Daily News*: 1991b).

The Patients' Rights Committee, lawyers, the police, many authors of newspaper articles and books on the subject of brain death, and even substantial numbers of the medical profession appear, therefore, to be publicly contesting the authority of transplant surgeons. What they usually cite as their principal cause for concern is a lack of trust in the medical teams who will make decisions about cases of brain death, because they believe that the pressure to retrieve organs will result in the process of dying being curtailed or even misdiagnosed. These critics are explicitly opposed to what they believe is the secrecy and arrogance of some members of the medical profession, and the vulnerability of patients and their families to exploitation in their hands. Many of these opponents of brain death argue strongly for informed consent at the same time. They also wish a frank disclosure and discussion of diagnoses with patients. Neither of those activities are routinely established in Japan. This contest apparently over the nature of scientific decisionmaking is, therefore in addition, a challenge to the hegemony of invested authority. The challengers characterize this authority as being exerted in a traditionally Japanese way, whereby subjects are rendered passive and are expected to comply to the medical regimen without question.

A national newspaper, the *Asahi Shinbun*, recently described the medical world as 'irritated' with government indecision over the issue. Doctors sense that their international reputations as outstanding surgeons are seriously threatened. At the annual meeting of the JMA held in 1991 in Kyoto, which I attended, two plenary sessions and several smaller panels were given over to brain death and organ transplants. The principal presenters of papers were physicians who had lived and worked for some time in the United States and who whilst there had practised transplant surgery. Apart from the scientific part of their presentations every one of them strongly asserted that Japanese medicine is suffering because of the national concern over brain death. They showed slides of themselves standing in surgical gowns, side by side with American transplant surgeons and happy patients who had recently received organ transplants. Such presentations at the JMA are the only time that I have heard more than the briefest of discussions in Japan about the feelings or rights of patients whose lives would be saved, however temporarily, by these procedures.

In the meantime doctors try to salvage what they can in the face of this intense debate by working to perfect artificial organs. They have also been experimenting with live liver donations from parents to children watched closely by the media (*Asahi Shinbun*: 1991). The most recent development to receive extensive Japanese television coverage was the participation by a Japanese doctor in a surgical team in America which transplanted a baboon liver to a human patient. Clearly, should this type of transplant become widely acceptable, it would circumvent the problem of brain death of a human donor entirely.

In concert with government, professional and media discussion is engaged in the most persistent search for national consensus (*kokuminteki goi*) among the Japanese public that has taken place on any subject. There have been 10 national surveys about brain death and organ transplants between 1983 and 1992. These surveys have demonstrated that the number of people who recognize brain death as the termination of life has increased from 29 per cent to approaching 50 per cent. In the most recent poll, there was a 79 per cent response rate of whom 72 per cent stated that they have an interest in the issues of organ transplants and brain death. As with all the previous surveys a paradox, perhaps indicating confusion, is evident in that more people approve of organ transplants from brain dead patients than those who accept brain death as the termination of life. In this most recent poll 55 per cent approved of organ transplants from brain dead patients, 14 per cent were opposed to such a possibility, and 30 per cent were undecided. Whilst only 51 per cent of men and 39 per cent of females agree that brain death is the end of life, nearly 50 per cent overall agreed that even if brain death is not formally recognized in Japan, a transplant would be acceptable if both the potential donor and his/her family have given consent (*Mainichi Shinbun*: 1991c).

Since it has been frequently reiterated that public consensus must be reached before brain death can be nationally recognized, the results of opinion polls are drawn on by those who are contesting brain death to support their argument. Nevertheless it appears that the whole exercise of repeatedly surveying the nation on this issue is essentially unproductive, a sentiment frequently voiced by the Japanese public, for the idea of trying to achieve a simple consensus on such an inflammatory subject is without meaning. Of particular importance is that those who do not accept brain death as the termination of life repeatedly state in the opinion polls that they take this position because they do not trust the medical profession.

In December 1990 Japanese national television (NHK) televized a three hour, Saturday evening prime time programme on the subject of brain death and organ transplants. This particular programme, which was not unique, was devised and moderated by the nationally recognized Tachibana Takashi, a journalist with the newspaper the *Yomiuri Shinbun*. It was divided into two parts. The first hour and a half was devoted to a film made largely in America about the harvesting and dispersal of organs on a nation wide basis. The second half of the programme was given over to a round table discussion between six 'experts', three for and three against the acceptance of brain death as the end of life. I have discussed this programme with several Japanese who saw it and, even those who are naturally sceptical about media presentations, responded that they thought it was a balanced discussion. In my opinion, however, it was clearly biased, but perhaps not intentionally so. Mr Tachibana is personally opposed to brain death, and has written numerous articles and two books to explain why he takes this position. Although he tried to remain neutral in moderating the programme, his position was clear (Tachibana: 1986).

To the background of sweet music, viewers are introduced at the beginning of the programme to a lively, beguiling Japanese child who was born from a brain dead mother and who, we are told symbolizes the fact that new life started from what is thought by some to be a dead body. The audience is then taken to North Carolina where a young man, badly damaged in a road accident, was pronounced brain dead and transported to another hospital where his heart was about to be removed when he "came back to life'. He lived for another six days before death was finally established. This section of the programme closes with a close-up of the large ornamental cross attached to the outside of the hospital, and the camera pans over a nearby graveyard filled with crosses and with a view of the hospital behind it.

In the next scene an American doctor states that it is difficult to diagnose brain death, that a clear legal definition is not possible. He indicates that if the guidelines are too lenient then one is in danger of misdiagnosing certain cases, but on the other hand with too stringent criteria many organs 'go to waste'. Later in the programme Willard Gaylin, a psychiatrist formally associated with the Hastings Center in New York, described the 'excitement' he experienced when he first realized that what he terms 'neomorts' could be used for testing new drugs, for medical students to dissect in place of using the bodies of poor people, and for 'recycling body parts into other people'. Earlier in the programme, he had vividly described the way in which 'neomorts' are still warm and breathing, but nevertheless legally dead. Yet another American doctor makes clear that in his opinion, not only brain dead bodies, but also people in so-called 'persistent vegetative states' will be recognized as dead in the near future. The camera then moves to a Japanese ward full of patients diagnosed as being in a 'persistent vegetative state' (*shokubutsu ningen*) and viewers are shown how some of these patients respond to human communication by subtle movements of their bodies and are told how, in another institution, 13 out of 30 patients in a persistent vegetative state made some significant recovery after constant intensive treatment, sometimes to the point of being able to speak again.

Together, these scenes and others like them in the programme, including several from Europe, give an impression that brain death is not easily diagnosed, and that in any case, brain dead patients are in some clear sense 'living'; that there is a continuum between brain death and other states, so that no easy boundary can be drawn. Thus a Western-style dichotomy cannot be made between the living and the dead unless one waits patiently for further proof in the form of whole body death, at which time vital organs such as the heart, liver, and lungs would no longer be fit for transplantation.

Viewers are then taken into a surgical unit in Florida where they see in graphic detail, and accompanied by a funereal-like sound track, the dismemberment of a young woman whose blond hair in one well angled shot is displayed through the drapes. They learn that 17 kinds of organs are taken from her, starting with the heart and ending up with large sections of bone, joint, and muscle tissue and are then shown several cartons of dismembered body parts stored in dry ice being wheeled out for computer organized distribution around the United States. The audience is told that, as a result of this seven hour 'operation', parts of this 21 year old will 'continue to live in 70 other people', and is then shown what is left of the body, tidied up by the nursing staff, ready for burial.

One other item which is raised as a major issue in this programme is the question of the sale of organs. No direct reference is made to the selling of organs in the United States, despite books and newspaper articles in Japanese occasionally citing such cases. Viewers are told about commercial trade in organs elsewhere. It is also noted that Brazilian children are taken illegally to Europe for possible slaughter and sale of their organs. A line of people in India waiting to sell one of their kidneys is shown, and it is indicated that they will receive the equivalent of five years' income.

At the end of the programme a professor at Tohuku University in Japan is introduced who, when he transplanted brain cells between mice, found that he could restore some of the brain functioning which he had previously destroyed in the recipient mice. This experiment indicates, viewers are told, that a brain dead person could perhaps be returned to life as a result of future developments in medicine. It is emphasized throughout this part of the programme that *because* death cannot be readily defined the brain death debate must inevitably be linked to ethics and religion. An implicit but clear contrast is set up between America, the pragmatic; the land of Christianity (symbolized by crosses on hospitals and in graveyards) where altruistic giving is part of the tradition, and where categorical decisions about death are reached quite easily, and Japan which being closer to nature, does not think in oppositional dichotomies, and thus is less willing to tinker with such important natural forces.

In the round table discussion which followed, the lawyer and two doctors arguing for the acceptance of brain death made a narrowly construed argument that brain death means the irreversible stoppage of brain functioning which can be rationally and systematically deduced with accuracy when certain procedures are correctly applied. Those making the argument for brain death returned again and again to universal scientific standards as the basis for decision making. They were explicit that what they termed 'emotional' arguments, apparently meaning references to values and cultural difference, should be kept out of the discussion. They noted that in America the donation of organs had been set up on a 'rational' basis in which people were free to refuse to participate.

In contrast, the three speakers opposed to the acceptance of brain death repeatedly stated that the religious background to the problem must be considered; that emotional matters and scientific theory should not be separated, but, on the contrary united; than an examination of the 'truth' must be accompanied by 'feelings as well as logic, and that the 'social concept' of death must be considered. One of the speakers taking this line of argument was the conservative philosopher

Umehara Takeshi, who, amongst the three opposition speakers against brain death criteria, characteristically made the most assertive statements. He pointed out that the 'Japanese people' dislike transplantations because they do not like 'unnatural' things. They have never in the past accepted extreme Chinese customs such as foot binding and the eunuch system. In a similar vein contemporary Japanese hate homosexuality and the use of drugs. He then laid the blame for the sorry state of 'the West' on René Descartes, for focusing attention on the brain as the centre of the living person. Nonetheless he went on to point out that humans everywhere are unique, rational beings. While 'Western modernism' makes 'us Japanese happy in one sense', he stated, at the same time it has 'destroyed our surroundings and nature'. If this discussion had taken place one month later, Professor Umehara would have been able to seize the opportunity to mention that a recent Japanese recipient of a kidney from a 'foreign' donor died of AIDS contracted from the transplanted organ.

A survey of the vast popular literature in Japanese on brain death shows that no simple ideological dichotomies can be drawn between those for and against its acceptance. While those of a conservative, traditionalist persuasion are unanimously opposed, they are joined by others who are politically left wing, such as the producer of the television programme, Mr Tachibana, and by many in the medical profession, both young and old, including some surgeons. Those politically active on behalf of handicapped and mentally ill people are also opposed to its acceptance. So too are many lawyers, those concerned about patients' rights and, apparently, the police. Advocates for acceptance of brain death include intellectual and professional people, among them physicians with Western training or experience. They are joined by nonprofessional people, including patient groups who are supporters of potential recipients of organs.

What is striking to an anthropologist is that it is mostly the culture and values of the Other which are scrutinized. Christian views are closely examined although concern about Judaism has not entered the debate. The question of rationality, and the idea of the brain as the centre of the body, and altruism and individuality are repeatedly discussed. But, despite a call to move beyond a discussion about scientific decision making, Japanese traditions and values are rarely examined explicitly. Among the more then 20 physicians whom I have interviewed on the subject, only two focused on cultural features in order to explain why the question of brain death is of such importance in contemporary Japan. One of them, a young surgeon who is opposed to the diagnosis of brain death, described *obon*, which is a major annual festival in which the dead return to earth and then after several days of ritual celebrations go back again in repose. Their departure is symbolized by thousands of tiny paper boats which are floated down stream. He asserted that these beliefs will continue to be a great significance to younger Japanese in the future. The other, a licensed physician who practises herbal medicine, discussed the concept of fate, and explained how life is understood in Japan as something larger than that of individual people; he emphasized that one's body is a parental gift, and that the lives of individuals belong, not to them, but to their family. However, these kinds of responses which draw heavily on Japanese cultural and philosophical tradition to buttress arguments against brain death are in the minority.

In considering the brain death debate it was striking how many features of Japanese culture could work against its acceptance as death, some of which have also been commented on by the Japanese anthropologist Emiko Namihira (1988). Among them the fact there has never been a philosophical thrust to separate mind and body is obviously significant. Further, the spiritual centre of the body is found in the metaphorical space known as the *kokoro* located in the region of the thorax, whereas the brain has little or no symbolic loading associated with it. But there are yet other facets of Japanese culture which contribute to the debate. The concept of the person in Japan has never been recognized as a unique bounded individual, but as someone residing at the centre of a network of obligations, so that personhood is constructed out-of-mind, beyond body, in the space of ongoing human relationships. The person in Japan is a dialogical creation, and what one does with and what is done to one's body is only in a limited way an individual affair. Moreover, ancestors remain as a presence in the Japanese cosmos, and for many people continue to participate in their daily lives. Even amongst those who have cast aside this tradition, many participate in the lengthy Buddhist orchestrated process over many years, which converts their dead relatives into ancestors. The idea of having a dismembered ancestor is associated with misfortune since their suffering in the other world can never be stopped. Moreover, Confucianism, the ethical tradition on which social life was grounded, for many centuries prohibited all tampering with dead bodies. Further, Shinto, the indigenous religion of Japan, regards all contact with death as ritually polluting. Of course many now categorically reject these 'old fashioned' beliefs and consider that any essentialist argument to the effect that Japanese culture effectively stops the acceptance of brain death would be entirely out of place. Nevertheless, cultural difference undoubtedly contributes to the present impasse whilst not being self-consciously examined in a more than perfunctory way.

The structure of hospital life in Japan also plays a role in the debate. Japanese families are deeply involved in the nursing of their dying relatives in many hospitals and they wash, lay-out and dress the corpse upon death. There is, therefore, much more familiarity than in many Northern European countries or North America with the process of dying and many Japanese are exceedingly alert as to how 'alive' a brain dead body appears to be. Sensitive about family concerns, most doctors are exceedingly reluctant to approach next-of-kin in Japan, especially women, to ask for permission to remove organs. It would be entirely inappropriate to pass this task to a junior doctor or a nurse. The result, is that on occasion doctors, having established in advance that relatives agree in principle to the donations of organs, simply proceed and remove kidneys without discussion of the brain death of the patient with the family.

The formal system of obligation upon which the exchange of gifts is based, although having no direct bearing on the definition of death, presents a major impediment to an easy acceptance of organ transplants in Japan. Gift giving is central in Japanese culture, and it is inevitably carried out within an established framework of ongoing reciprocity. Receiving an organ donated anonymously is not easy to accept, for the question of repayment and reciprocity looms large. Furthermore despite a comprehensive socialized health care system, gift giving to physicians is an established part of the system whereby doctors are encouraged to do their best for patients. There is thus a public fear that many organs will not be freely donated or will be bought and sold.

Of all these factors, this last is the only one which is considered with any regularity in a discussion of what it is about Japanese society which inhibits the acceptance of brain death and the routinization of organ transplants. Part of the reason is that there is a natural reluctance by Japanese to resort to 'tradition' to explain their world today. Both Emiko Namihira and the author have been chided for focusing too much attention on the 'uniqueness' of Japan, a position usually reserved for Japanese nationalists and the extreme right. Nevertheless, despite the dangerous direction this path potentially takes, it seems unwise to abandon a cultural thesis entirely as an explanation for at least part of the resistance to brain death. Such a position is reinforced by the way that the culture of the Other is being actively appropriated by so many Japanese to account for North American and European acceptance of the use of brain death with apparently little hesitation.

In the NHK television programme, Mr Tachibana pointed out that when considering a subject as difficult as that of death, it is important to examine how other countries have managed this issue. This plea calls to mind the Iwakura mission more than 100 years ago sent to Europe and America after the formal ending of 250 years of self-imposed isolated feudalism in Japan. Its task was to examine the democratic process, the school system, armed forces, legal and medical systems, treatment of women, and so on in various countries. Members of the Japanese Diet had previously expressed an opinion similar to that of Mr Tachibana, and one of the mandates of the special Committee was to travel widely, not only throughout Japan but also in Europe, America, Australia, and Thailand in order to study the situation in those countries. This Committee was therefore explicitly requested to reach an agreement about what would be best for Japan in light of a long and close scrutiny of the Other.

Of all the countries which they visited, the one which captured most media attention was Denmark, because brain death was accepted there only in July 1990, and until that time patients went abroad for transplants, as currently do some Japanese. Prior to its acceptance in Denmark, there were over 200 public hearings in that country and considerable government publicity on the subject. This experience led some members of the Committee to state that, despite all that had been published so far in Japanese, there had still not been enough public discussion. The Committee was also impressed with the trust shown in doctors, particularly in the European countries which they visited, a situation in contrast to that in Japan.

Allowing ones' dead relatives to be cut up for organ donation is genuinely repulsive to many Japanese. However, others are keen to be allowed to donate parts of their own body or of their close relatives to save the lives of others. Clearly major concerns for both those for and against organ donation centre on reports published with great regularity on an unprofessional medical world. The section on the NHK programme which showed Indians selling their kidneys, and the blatant fantasy which has appeared in more than one article in Japanese about poor black Americans selling their dead children to hospitals (Amano: 1987) reveals a deep seated fear that in Japan, should brain death be accepted, the buying and selling of organs will be established rather rapidly as a matter of course. Again and again, people interviewed, including physicians, have made unsolicited statements to the effect that doctors are not to be trusted in Japan. What passes for *omoiyari* – sympathy and consideration – is unqualified paternalism, and medical ethics have no meaning because very few people seriously question the power of the medical profession, who essentially look after their own interests. Medicine used to be thought of as a benevolent art: *i wa jin jitsu nari*, today everyone knows the pun in which medicine is now characterized as a money making art, *i wa kin jitsu nari*.

What is slowly being recognized is that whilst brain death is a culturally sensitive topic, it is no longer the definition of death, nor the remaking of the human body which is of prime importance. Many believe that brain death will be made legally acceptable in Japan in the near future, and that inspection trips abroad and the search for national consensus are placatory exercises before organ transplants are legalized despite the probability that few organs will be donated. It has been suggested that if the first Japanese heart transplant had not led to a legal battle, the entire brain death debate may never have entered the public domain and decision makers in the medical profession would simply have proceeded unilaterally in this area, as happened in North America. However, because the contest over the definition of death captured media attention, and the public became involved, the medical world has been exposed to public scrutiny in a way never before experienced. The media and Japanese citizens have thus taken on this 'secret society'. It is being attacked frontally in relation to many aspects of its current practices, ranging from a resistance to informed consent, to taking out uteri on a large scale for profit. At one level opposition to brain death is indeed a flamboyant expression of a major ideological struggle over relationships of power in modern Japan. While North America is cited as a negative example in the debate over brain death, simultaneously, it is drawn upon by critics as a model to emulate in relation to the handling of power. Japan in turn is denigrated as feudalistic and backward by comparison. This particular contest over death also reveals, as does another topical debate about the 'aging society', that in recent years Europe, particularly Scandinavia, has emerged in the Japanese consciousness as a significant Other for possible emulation, to be used to promote an ideological position which favours the fostering of social equality which is less 'individualistic' than that of America.

Contemporary Japan, like North America, is in theory a rational and secular society. Appellations such as 'tradition', 'culture' and 'religion' suggest superstition and pre-modern sentimentality. However, until recently Japan, although not outwardly espousing convergence theories of modernization, has nevertheless thought of itself as 'catching up'. This position has now changed. Japan for the first time is being pressed into a leadership role in the modern world order. There is an increasing recognition that there is more than one form of modernization, and that much can be learnt from the distinctive features of the Japanese case. The result is that the Japanese situation continues to be juxtaposed to that of the West and is repeatedly described by many commentators inside and outside the country as 'different'.

Historically, Confucianism, although mandated by Heaven, was predominantly a secular and highly rational system of ethics which, whilst imported from China in the sixth century, failed to take a dominant position in Japanese society until the sixteenth century. After this time it held sway for more than 250 years. Although both Buddhism and Shinto have always been powerful religious forces, the secular tradition of NeoConfucian behavioural norms was the dominant ideology both for political and daily life until the end of the last century. Its stamp is still very evident in many areas of Japanese society. It is safe to say that the majority of mature Japanese intuitively believe at present that the ethic of individualism has gone too far in North America. Deification of the individual was never part of the process of secularization in Japan. Society was deified, and hierarchical social mores inevitably took, and usually continue to take, precedence over individual needs. The very notion of individual rights is tainted with an aura of selfishness, and the idea of a thoroughly autonomous individual is patently absurd to most Japanese (as indeed it is for many 'Westerners').

The present dilemma for liberal minded thinkers in Japan is how to dispose of the remnants of patriarchal and patronage thinking without drawing on a language which single mindedly pursues the entrenchment of individual autonomy and rights. Further, it is how to create a meaningful social contract in late modernity which follows neither the authoritarianism of Confucianism nor the perceived anomie of individualism. It is in this context that the argument about brain death is taking place, and, as in the West, it is an overwhelmingly secular argument in which representatives of religious organizations are, for the most part, remarkably absent (Hardacre: ms). The debate is essentially about legitimization of scientific knowledge, the status of the medical profession, and the public interest. Scientific progress, Japan's image as an advanced society, and the value or otherwise or tradition are implicit in the argument, but debates on individual and family suffering are largely pushed to one side. So too is any serious exploration of subjective feelings, the sanctity of the body, human decency, the limits of scientific exploration, which are effectively displaced onto the Other. These issues are transformed into an ambivalent and ideological portrayal of what is purportedly happening outside Japan.

At its most abstract level, therefore, the current angst in Japan over brain death is a manifestation of the ceaseless, restless, contradictory debate about Japan and the West; tradition and modernity. This is not to suggest that a good deal of genuine passion does not go into contested meanings of death. However, this debate, partly because it is framed in the language of difference, has fanned the flames for further, painful comparisons which reach beyond medical procedures. At stake are questions of progress, internationalization, scientific and technological expertise, the relationship of the State, professional bodies, and the media, to society at large, and to individuals. The posing of these questions is in turn a manifestation of the struggle by people from a whole range of political persuasions to create an ethics for modern and postmodern Japan which is not simply a copy of those in the West. In entering the debate, traditionalists find themselves rubbing shoulders with those who are promoting further reform towards social equality and the empowerment of individuals. Physicians who believe that their authority should not be subjected to questioning find themselves in the same camp as the mentally impaired. Patients' rights advocates who are striving for more autonomy for the person in the street find themselves supporting the police as they extend the heavy hand of the law. Meanwhile little is heard from those immediately concerned with the results of transplantation, that is patients and their families, whether they be potential donors or recipients.

One obvious result of this ongoing debate about death is that there is in Japan a large number of people who are informed on the complexity of the problem. They contribute to national discussion and will presumably influence the course it takes. If and when transplants from brain dead bodies become acceptable, people will have a sense that they have participated in the decision making process. In contrast, in North America there was almost no public discussion about the redefinition of death. A decision was reached unilaterally by an Ad Hoc Committee of selected physicians in 1968. Now organ transplants are thoroughly routinized and a national computerized organ bank has been established. Several European countries find themselves in a similar position. The discussion today in the United States is of 'rewarded gifting', and 'organ wastage', signs of the urgent need to procure more and more organs in a steady move towards the large scale commodification of human parts. There is little discussion about the flow of organs from the poor to the rich, from the Third World to the First World, and even less of possible atrocities involved, despite documentation by Amnesty International. Leon Kass has described this process as a 'coarsening of sensibilities and attitudes', and adds 'there is a sad irony in our biomedical project, accurately anticipated in Aldous Huxley's *Brave New World*: We expend enormous energy and vast sums of money to preserve and prolong bodily life, but in the process our embodied life is stripped of its gravity and much of its dignity. This is, in a word, progress as tragedy' (Kass: 1992). It is usually assumed, moreover, that in a thoroughly secular society with a monolithic tradition, there is no need for an 'emotional' discussion about death. This is patently absurd. Not only are the sentiments of families of dying people ignored, so too are the feelings of health care professionals, especially nurses who are the only personnel to stay through the whole procedure of dismemberment. Nor is it established if the diagnosis of brain death is indeed completely reliable; I have been told by experts that it is 'in the hands of competent individuals'. Is this good enough? There are very few reports about the immuno- suppressant drugs which organ recipients must take for the rest of their lives which may put them at higher risk from cancer and various infectious diseases. We hear almost nothing of how it is to live with someone else's heart inside of one. We cannot now reverse the process. However it seems that some prolonged and painful self-reflection is in order and there may well be something to be learned from the Japanese case.

REFERENCES

Amano, K. (1987), 'Nôshi o Kangaeru, Zôki Ishoku to no Kanren no Naka de' (Thoughts on Brain Death in Connection with Organ Transplants). *Gekkan Naashingu* xvv(xiii), pp. 1949–53

Asahi Shinbun (1989), ' "Jin Ishoku o Chûkai" to Sagi'. April 23rd

Asahi Shinbun (1991), '14 Reimoku no Seitai Kan Shoku'. March 16th

Faludi, Susan (1991), *Backlash: The Undeclared War Against American Women*, Crown Publishers Inc., New York

Hardacre, Helen (ms), 'The Response of Buddhism and Shintô to the Issue of Brain Death and Organ Transplants'

Kass, Leon (1992), 'Organs for sale? Propriety, Property and the price of progress', *The Public Interest* April, pp. 65–84

Mainichi Daily News (1984), 'Organs Removed from Women Without Consent.' December 24th

Mainichi Daily News, (1991a), 'Kidney Transplant from Brain-Dead Man Revealed'. May 30th

—— (1991b), 'Bar Mixes Brain Death Criteria'. September 21st

—— (1991a), 'Cover-Up Suspected in First Heart Transplant'. March 31st

—— (1991b), 'Family Not Told of Donor's Brain- Death'. May 31st

—— (1991c), '55 per cent Approve of Transplants from Brain-Dead.' October 16th

Nakayama, Taro (1989), *Nôshi to Zôki Ishoku*, Saimaru Shuppansha, Tokyo

Namihira, E. (1988), *Nôshi, Zôki Ishoku, Gan Kokuchi*, Fukubu Shoten, Tokyo

Nihon Keizai Shinbun (1992), ' "Nôshi Ishoku" Michisuji nao Futômei'. January 23rd

Tachibana, Takeshi (1986), *Nôshi (Brain Death)*, Chûôkôronsha, Tokyo

12

What is power? How is decision? The heart has its reasons

RONALD FRANKENBERG

FORE AND AFTERWORD

What follows is in fact a prolegomenon to an empirical study of narratives of heart patients and their surgeons on decision-taking processes in a famous heart surgery unit.

The first direction of the main study would be to explore the proposition that *informed consent is improbable* because, while concepts may be shared in the present context of interaction, the context of future action is too divergent. To the ill sufferer, self-perceived, heart disease is a fuzzily defined incident in the flow of life experience in the incarnate body at the heart of which s/he lives; to the surgeon, the sight is of a sick patient's corporeal body laid open or laying him/herself open to end a bounded episode of sickness by the excision and/or replacement of diseased somatic tissue.

The second proposition to be tested is that *informed refusal is impossible* (Hill 1992) because the mutual understandings of patients, nurses and surgeons are mediated by 'boundary objects ... a class of object that is used by members from different social worlds, often being very differently perceived by members of those worlds. Boundary objects are both plastic enough to adapt to local needs and constraints, yet robust enough to maintain a common identity across sites, times or social worlds' (Bowker and Star 1990 p. 6; see also Star and Griesemer 1989; Star 1988; and King and Star 1990). It is argued that the process of surgical treatment for heart disease may be seen as such an object behind which are concealed both differences and similarities of perception. These are generated by unshared formal training and shared publicly mediated experience. It is not, of course, that the patients alone have embodied knowledges, but the language of different actors is used to reduce embodied knowledges to superficially similar but profoundly different shared views.

MEDICAL TECHNOLOGY AND LANGUAGES OF THE BODY: AN ARGUMENTAL COLLAGE IN THREE MOVEMENTS

I Pre-Text

(a) Totalities can only be conveyed in an occult manner. God's name is capable of being addressed in language but not of being uttered in language. *For only its fragmentariness renders language utterable.* The 'true' language cannot be uttered, just as the absolutely concrete cannot be realised.

(Gershon Sholem, *Ten Unhistorical Aphorisms on Kabbalah* in Biale, 1985 p. 86, cited by Handelman 1991 p. 86, author's italics)

as against

The aim of the philosophy of language (I caricature, of course) is usually not so much to describe, as to purify natural languages to preserve the possibility of communicative and referential uses, to save language for science. Even when the aim is only to describe, as in the theory of speech acts, another, underlying object soon appears to preserve the possibility of scientific discussion and progress by defending a conception of meaning as intentional and dialogue as cooperative.

Against this, I have tried to argue that linguistic exchange is a locus for relations of power, that far from occurring in a cooperative vacuum it depends on historical and linguistic conjuncture and often involves agonistic strategy and tactics. This, of course, implies a theory of the subject of subjectification as subjection, that is incompatible with the subject as centre of consciousness and control which cooperation and intentional meaning require.

(Jean-Jacques Lecercle, *The Violence of Language*, London: Routledge 1990 p. 267)

(b) Today we know quite well this experience of estrangement, for the distance which separates our knowledge of the world from our experience of it has only increased. Between my body, which I know in living my life with others, and the body of medical knowledge, or between the atomic structure of matter and the things of the world which I sense with my body, there lies an immeasurable distance, and in most respects each of us remains a stranger to these constructed realities. We *know*, often in fine detail, the world we have imagined and dreamed, the world we have created, but we cannot experience it. No matter how hard I may try, for example, to *experience* my sight of a beautiful sunrise as the impact of electromagnetic radiation upon the retinas of my eyeballs where complex electrochemical reactions take place transforming physical stimuli into physiological events, I am doomed to fail. I may succeed, of course, in transforming all of these physical and physiological processes into visual displays which I can see, but the lines and patterns observed on monitor screens are quite clearly *not* the same thing as the sight of a glorious sunrise. And indeed, were I to claim in all honesty and sincerity that I could *experience* that sunrise as a conjunction of physical stimuli and physiological events, I would be judged insane. This is the epitome of estrangement, for the very same world created by a self in distance is judged both to be *real*, the way the world is, a complex of physico-chemical relations transformed into neuro-chemical events, and *illusion*. Small wonder, then, that in this estrangement we should begin to lose our way.

(Romanyshin 1989 p. 68)

(c) It is, in the words of the art critic Charles Wentinck, a body which has become 'an almost inhuman abstraction, further removed from nature than at any other moment in history'. It is a body enshelled, a body where 'All the natural activities – of hearing, breathing, speaking and making gestures are ... replaced by technical functions', a body closed in upon itself and insulated from the world. A key issue for our age is to understand the ways *we are* this body. It is a key issue because the way in which we understand and treat our bodies is a reflection of the way we understand and treat the world.

(Romanyshin 1989 p. 103)

(d) Of course the physicians who have taken care of me, the surgeons who have operated on me, have been able to have direct experience with the body which I myself do not know. I do not disagree with them. I do not claim that I lack a brain, a heart, or a stomach. But it is most important to choose the order of our bits of knowledge. So far as the physicians have had any experience with my body, it was with my body, in the midst of the world as it is for others. My body as it is for me does not appear to me in the midst of the world. Of course during a radioscopy I was able to see the picture of my vertebrae on a screen, but I was outside in the midst of the world. I was apprehending a wholly constituted object as 'a this' amongst other 'thises', and it was only through a reasoning process that I referred it back to being mine: it was much more my property than my being.

(Sartre, *Being and Nothingness* pp. 279–80 quoted in Taussig 1992 p. 85)

(e) Oh, ho, ho, ho, ho! What the devil is this? Do you call this ordure, ejection, excrement, evacuation, *dejecta*, fecal matter, *egesla, copros, scatos,* dung, crap, turds? Not at all. not at all: it is but the fruit of the shittim tree, 'Selah! Let us drink.'

(Rabelais, *Works*, Harmondsworth: Penguin, Book 4 Chapter 67)

Here we find twelve synonyms for excrement, from the most vulgar to the most scientific. At the end it is described as a tree, something rare and pleasant. And the tirade concludes with an invitation to drink, which in Rabelaisian imagery means to be in communion with truth.

(Bakhtin 1984 p. 175)

(f) After the departure of a lover, the narrator (she?) finds the bed empty even when she herself is in it. She cycles to the library and goes to the medical books. She writes:

I became obsessed with anatomy. If I could not put Louise out of my mind I would drown myself in her. Within the clinical language, through the dispassionate view of the sucking, sweating, greedy, defecating self, I found a love-poem to Louise. I would go on knowing her, more intimately than the skin, hair and voice that I craved. I would have her plasma, her spleen, her synovial fluid. I would recognise her even when her body had long since fallen away.'

The multiplication of cells by mitosis occurs throughout the life of the individual. It occurs at a more rapid rate until growth is complete. thereafter new cells are formed to replace those which have died. Nerve cells are a notable exception. When they die they are not replaced.

'In the secret places of her thymus gland Louise is making too much of herself. Her faithful biology depends on regulation but the white T-cells have turned bandit. They don't obey the rules. They are swarming into the bloodstream, overturning the quiet order of spleen and intestine. In the lymph nodes they are swelling with pride. It used to be their job to keep her body safe from enemies on the outside. They were her immunity, her certainty against infection. Now they are the enemies on the inside. The security forces have rebelled. Louise is the victim of a *coup*.

'Will you let me crawl inside you, stand guard over you, trap them as they come at you? Why can't I dam their blind tide that filthies your blood? Why are there no lock gates on the portal vein? The inside of your body is innocent, nothing has taught it fear. Your artery canals trust their cargo, they don't check the shipments in the blood. You are full to overflowing but the keeper is asleep and there's murder going on inside. Who comes here? Let me hold up my lantern. It's only the blood; red cells carrying oxygen to the heart, thrombocytes making sure of proper clotting. The white cells, B and T types, just a few of them as always whistling as they go.

'The faithful body has made a mistake. This is no time to stamp the passports and look at the sky. Coming up behind are hundreds of them. Hundreds too many, armed to the teeth for a job that doesn't need doing. Not needed? With all that weaponry? Here they come, hurtling through the bloodstream trying to pick a fight. There's no one to fight but you Louise. You're the foreign body now.'

(Winterson 1992 pp. 126–7)

II Con-Text

Social science is itself a technology practised in and for society. It too has advanced from stylus on wax through pen on paper to tape recorder, scanner, video camera and word processor. It aspires to the God-like power of knowing the end of a thing while it is still beginning. No wonder it seems to many to have merely re-created Babel, the real link between postmodern architecture and the social theories that bear its name.

Obviously medicine has also always been and always will be a technology practised on and by the body. Hippocrates, Galen and Maimonides were as much technologists of the body as the Harefield or Cleveland Cardiac surgery *equips*. What is now feared, and what we mean by high technology, is that while in the past the sensations of the organic body determined the nature (*sic*) of technology now the perceptions of mechanistic technology determines the culture of the body.

Armstrong (1983, 1985) following and developing Foucault, drew our attention to three main aspects of modern medicine in relation to the body: its exercise of power over the bodies of its patients and the control of the patient's time and the disposition of his/her body in space which aids this exercise of power. Thus as the practice of medicine became more technical the sphere of practice of the primary health care physician, in Britain, moved from the patient's home to his own, from there to the purpose-built annexe and finally to the health centre. Similarly with increasing technology in long term care the acute life threatened patient was moved at least temporarily into hospital and the Intensive Care Unit (ICU) or Coronary Care Unit (CCU) perhaps to be discharged, carrying with them embodied hospital space in the form of pacemaker, mechanical valve or the like. Thus while high technology may involve segregation in space and time, higher still may make either liberation or, as it were, parole possible. Electronic and chemical technology have made the liberal dreams of decarceration for patients and prisoners a conservative reality. The progressive confinement of the body as patient in a space and for a time controlled by the institutions of medicine runs parallel with the insertion or implantation within the patient of the mechanical naturomimetic artefacts of technological medicine.

John Jacobs (1988) argues that since the patient loses expertise, control and the possibility of informed and therefore genuine choice in the move from primary through secondary to tertiary care, the application of medicine becomes more 'pure' in a sense which I read to be that criticised by Scheper Hughes and Lock (1987) in their now classic paper on the mindful body (which is another prolegomenon!). There they suggest the existence of at least three bodies. The first, the body social, was noticed initially, in what might be called a pre-analytical way, by the French sociologist follower of Durkheim, Marcel Mauss (1973) when in 1935 he drew attention to the differing ways in which the French and the English used their bodies in marching, in swimming, in digging and in all other ways. What he called the 'techniques of the body' shared a common (he called it natural) productive, instrumental, end in locomotion or in achieving work, but an expressive (cultural/social) difference so that to the initiated observer there was no doubt who was French or English. He argued that psychological determination in individual terms was a mere cog in transmission and that each new generation was taught or imitated, but not quite exactly, the customary ways of bodily doing of their immediate forebears.

Within French sociology/anthropology, Bourdieu took up his predecessor's term for this, 'habitus', and developed and refined it to portray the personal bodily attitude to the world shared to some extent by all French people, for example, but differentiated by class and status, gender and education. Those with the right to rule enjoyed not only knowledge in the cognitive sense but also correct deportment. Those with the duty to obey showed if not the fixed mark of Cain at least the demeanour of Adam after the fall or of the incessant humbling activity of grinning Martha. Looked at from the individuals' viewpoint, their cultural capital was embodied knowledge not just of what to say but how to express it both in words and in other bodily actions and products. Looked at from the point of view of society at large the institutions of the social world were reflected in the way bodies worked and played.

Mary Douglas (1970, 1973) combined the outcome of this Durkheimian genealogy with another of the same lineage but descending in a different line through Bernstein's analysis of linguistic codes and the principles of classification and hierarchy. She suggests ways in which social change, mediated through stylistic concordance on all channels (movement, dress, performance of bodily functions), leads to the transmission and control of bodily behaviour from, for example, the upright gait and clipped speech and moustaches of the officers of the Gardes Républicains or Household Brigade to the carefully modified shagginess of hair and posture which literally marks the intellectual and/or aesthete. This very brief discussion has already implied a partial shift to Scheper-Hughes and Lock's second body, the body politic. For it is clear that the interaction of the social and the body of each individual member of society is not innocent of considerations of asymmetrical power. Foucault (amongst others) has cogently argued both the social necessity of a state controlling the bodies of its members and the divers ways in which, at different times, persons have been variously coerced, surveilled, constrained, and con-scienced to control the members of their bodies. Modern medicine, has as it happens, grown and been developed within the interstices of these discontinuous changes in the ways and scale of the exercise of power. Interventions in the workings of the body perceived as sick, including the classification of signs and symptoms and the isolation and naming of diseases and syndromes are cultural and conjunctural products, specific to time, place and the respective positions of internal and external observers. The same is true of perceptions of the body seen as normal, in despite of or rather through the observations of biological science as Laqueur (1990) has demonstrated for the history of the sexual apparatus.

Marx was famously translated as having said that man makes his own history but does not make it out of whole cloth (Marx 1951), and another lineage of French thinkers this time out of Merleau-Ponty have argued the same for the bodies of both main genders. The lived body, the Leib (Ots 1990) or mindful body, creates itself within the cultural framework, i.e. the processes of self creation of its others, by which it finds itself encompassed. Romanyshyn (1989) from whom I have mined two of the six pre-texts above points to the simultaneous inventions of perspective and the corpse. He shows how the under-standing of the body politic of the principality on the one hand and of the bodies of its citizens on the other was distanced and made reliable, replicatable and reproducible at the same time as the particu-larities and specificities of their being in the world was distorted and simplified. He does this by contrasting a view of Florence before the invention of perspective with one painted shortly afterwards. In the first we feel that we might well bump into the walls or into fellow human beings. We can almost smell what Italians call in contrast to the odour of sanctity, *humanitas*. In the second we are distanced. The buildings are seen in orderly ranks and too far away to know if they are even inhabited; the first stage of a process that was to lead to aerial photography and the Registrar-General's classifications. He puts these in apposition with two portraits of anatomists alongside the human body. In the first the scientist embraces and looks at the body whole and little detail is seen within it; in the second, Vesalius is depicted displaying the interior of one dismembered arm and stands beside it, holding but not looking at it. He looks at us, little Jack Horner who has just discovered the plum. He has destroyed the perduring living body as the basis of life and medicine and invented the corpse, as well as the more somatic fragment. He has laid an uncertain but enduring foundation for the lay/professional contradiction within health care (including that between nurse and doctor): '7H nurses did not give post mortem care to dead bodies. Instead they cared for patients they knew both before and after death' (Wolf 1988 p. 68). We must assume that ancient doctors, like relatives at most times, the religious and the modern nurses cited above, saw their patients as moving from living to dead rather than from body incarnate to waste matter. Nevertheless it is probably fair to recognise that what we might call corporeal knowledge was made possible by this distancing and a certain lack of respect. Modern medicine, even before its high technology phase, advanced knowledge of the corporeal body by specialising minutely on its several parts and the systems related to them. This we might call the *somatic* body. The achievements of modern medicine, and they are, of course, considerable, depend in the first instance in distancing the clinical observer/ practitioner from the body incarnate which is reduced to the body corporeal. Then the body corporeal is itself dismembered into its somatic components. These latter are clearly often, for minutes, months or even years, mechanically substitutable.

Within the phenomenological tradition, Bologh (1979, 1981) has argued that for medicine in its strictest most scientific form, it was not necessary to recognise that the patient had a creative mind merely that s/he might have an obstructive will. On the other hand in a society based on, and impressed by electronically controlled machine technology, medicine does more than cure. It demonstrates understanding and definition of brute nature and an ability successfully to combat its vagaries. Because of its sophisticated technology, tertiary care gives pleasure in and hope to society, even if it does not always give comfort. Jacobs (1988) cites Hirschman's distinction in the field of all consumer durables, domestic as well as medical, between comfort providers and pleasure providers.

Pleasure is the experience of travelling from discomfort to comfort while the latter is achieved at the point of arrival. Hence a contradiction between pleasure and comfort; for pleasure to be experienced comfort must be sacrificed temporarily. Thus society permits and wants medicine to devote, 'extraordinary resources to dealing with extraordinary manifestations of illness. The resources, for example, devoted to organ transplants are out of all proportion to any other benefit society gains' (Jacobs 1988 p. 59). It must also be admitted that it is social 'scientists' who, having gifted the title of biomedicine to those who practise it, now question whether they should allow them to keep it! Honest doctors and philosophers, however modern(ist), have readily admitted, even boasted, in anecdote and memoir that a lot of medicine is based on hunch and experience rather than on biology. Even more fundamental, while patients bring their intact or damaged whole bodies to surgery or hospital, as I have just argued, doctors are beneficially selective about the parts to which they give their attention. At any point of time the medical gaze is focused on the part rather than the whole and on the present or the short term past with an eye to the future (prognosis and treatment) rather than on the aeons of biological evolution or the nanoseconds of molecular biology. The medical view of the body differs from the biological in the limitations of its extension over bodyspace and over time. This necessarily limited but important view, a focused gaze, I have called *somatic* to distinguish it from the broader biological *corporeal*. Finally to describe roughly the mindful body without lending credence to a Cartesian dichotomy I have introduced the term body *incarnate* to try to suggest the feeling of human wholeness which for many is, or ought to be the normative state. Judith Monks and I (1994) in examining the autobiographies of persons with multiple sclerosis believe that we found evidence of the emic use of body in all three ways and Ots (1990) in phenomenologically based recent work on Chinese traditional medicine uses the German terms *Körper* and *Leib* which I have borrowed to indicate the last two.

The conceptual divorce between science and art, mind and body, reality and image, reason and emotion which is traced back to Aristotle through Plato and from Plato through Descartes to high modernism enters into medical praxis through the mechanism (or organicism?) I have just outlined. Through tragic, because inevitable, necessity,

medicine has had to abandon the unspeakable and unthinkable totality for the describable, analysable and therefore thinkable manipulation of body fragments which provide a major taxonomic framework
for disease and diagnosis and especially for surgical specialties.
Patients however remain within a discourse dominated by *illness* in
which symptoms are seen as continuous with and related to other
troubles. The patients' differential diagnosis of illness leads to choice
of resource provider: doctor, lawyer, lover, policeman or friend; the
doctors' differential diagnosis of disease leads primarily to choice of
body pathology: heart disease, brain damage, liver malfunction. It is
an artefact of the history of modern medicine and the division of
specialties within it that this last series of diagnoses leads to a secondary choice of specifically qualified resource persons in turn. The differences between sufferers and healers are not therefore in my view,
merely of varying explanatory models (see Kleinman 1980 but compare Kleinman 1988 and also for a use of explanatory models within
the spirit of what I am here arguing, Farmer 1988, 1990, 1992) but
of quite different fields of discourse with quite different views of the
nature of knowledges and their interconnections. Doctors seek consent for procedures within one discourse: patients give it within
another. They do not necessarily disagree about what should be the
outcome even though their mutual misunderstanding may outweigh
their mutual understanding.

It is for this reason that some writers have added *sickness* to the
concepts of the illness experienced by the patient and the disease
treated by the doctor. As Gerry Stimson and Barbara Webb (1975)
long ago argued in Britain and Eliot Freidson in the United States,
consultations are usually, if not always, negotiations in which the
discourses of partially conflicting realities are superficially reconciled.
This has now almost become a cliché in primary health care, although
in secondary and tertiary care differentials of knowledge and power
still mask its realities. I have defined both sickness and medical anthropology in terms of *cultural performance*. This is a ludic metaphor which
has its roots in the seventeenth and eighteenth centuries'operating
and lecture theatres (Stafford 1991) and which is intended to imply
an audience which is in no way disinterested. The doctor-patient
interaction is neither symmetrical or socially neutral either in its heart-
lands (*sic*) or further afield (Comaroff 1985, Vaughan 1991: McLeod
and Lewis 1988). This has obvious implications for the so-called compliance problem, more properly perhaps called patient choice; for
health promotion; for the ethics of individual and social decision

taking not least in the area of ceasing treatment; and, most importantly, because of their role as interpreters between doctorspeak and
patientspeak, for the daily practice of nurses (Gadow 1980; Lawlor
1991;Benner 1994). The texts that follow illustrate these differing
discourses in relation to heart disease.

III Texts

Angina: A novel view (feelings, continuities, syntheses)

The sky is a blank redness out of which Pru's factual Ohio voice falls
with a concerned intonation . . .

The redness pulses with pain spaced like ribs, stripes of pain with
intervals of merciful nothingness between them. Very high up, slowly,
an airplane goes over, dragging its noise behind it . . . He lies there like
a jelly fish washed up, bulging tremblingly full of desire for its lost
element. Another complicated warmish thing, with fingers is touching
his wrist, feeling his pulse. First aid must be part of Gregg's job. To
assist him in his diagnosis Harry volunteers. 'Sorry to be such a crump,
I had this terrific desire to lie down.'

'You keep lying there, Mr Angstrom,' Gregg says, sounding suddenly
loud and crisp and a touch too authoritative, like his father adding up
the golf scores, 'We're going to get you to the hospital . . .'

In his red blind world this is such a relief he opens his eyes. He sees
Judy [his small grandchild] standing huge and sun haloed above him'
(Updike 1990 pp. 116–17)

Angina: a nursing text (signs, discontinuities, analyses)

Angina Pectoris.'The classic indication of impaired circulation to the
myocardium is a distinctive type of chest pain called *angina pectoris.* The
pain signifies insufficient oxygenation (*ischemia*) of the myocardium; it
occurs when the oxygen demands of the myocardium exceed the
capacity of the coronary circulation to supply oxygen. In other words,
angina represents a signal from the heart, indicating that the myocardium is not receiving sufficient oxygen to meet its needs at the moment.
Because the angina pectoris is usually the key to the diagnosis of CHD,
it is essential to understand its clinical features.

Site of Pain. The pain of myocardial ischaemia is located most often
directly under the center of the breastbone. it may radiate from this
substernal location to both sides of the chest, the left or right arm, the
neck the jaws, or the shoulders and upper back. in some instances
the pain occurs only at these latter sites without a substernal component;
this pattern however, is much less common than central chest pain.

Quality of Pain. The discomfort is usually described as pressure, tightness, or constriction within the chest. Some patients place a clenched fist against the sternum to characterize the tight, constricting nature of the sensation. Although angina generally lasts for only a few minutes (as described below), the pain is steady and is not influenced by breathing, breath holding, or change in body position. This constancy of the pain is a characteristic aspect of angina and is often more significant than other descriptive qualities (e.g. burning, pressure or 'indigestion').' [Chapter 1 continues with paragraphs headed: Occurrence of Pain, Duration of Pain, Relief of Pain, Diagnosis of Angina Pectoris, Exercise (Stress) Testing, Radionucleide Studies, Coronary Arteriography, stable and Variant Angina Pectoris, Intermediate Coronary Syndrome (Unstable Angina) and Acute Myocardial Infarction which is introduced and then elaborated in Chapter 2].

(Meltzer, Pinneo and Kitchell 1983)

Angina: a medical text (historical, comprehensive, contextualised, cautiously definitive but magisterial)

Synonyms. Angina of effort; Heberden's angina

Definition. Angina pectoris was described by Heberden in 1768, but its relation to coronary disease was not appreciated until the present century. Angina pectoris is essentially a clinical syndrome of characteristic chest pain produced by increased cardiac work and relieved by rest. The underlying cause is occlusive disease of the coronary arteries, which is mostly atheroma, sometimes syphilitic coronary ostial stenosis, and very rarely coronary embolism or congenital anomalies of the coronary vessels. Cardiac pain identical with angina pectoris may also be caused by aortic stenosis and less commonly aortic incompetence; it also occurs in patients with severe pulmonary hypertension and rarely in pulmonary stenosis. Anaemia, if severe, may cause cardiac pain, but rarely of the severity met with in coronary atheroma. Angina pectoris may be associated with myxoedema, rarely with thyrotoxicosis and frequently with diabetes mellitus, and in these conditions is the underlying cause. [Continues with a page on clinical features a paragraph each on the electrocardiogram and other investigations, a page follows on each of diagnosis, treatment and treatment of underlying causes before it too moves on to myocardial infarction.]

(Scott 1973 Section 8 pp. 772–6)

Catheterisation: a nursing text

Balloon Dilatation of Coronary Arteries. The newest approach to the treatment of symptomatic CHD involves dilatation of narrowed segments of coronary arteries by means of a small balloon catheter inserted into the obstructed vessel by way of a peripheral artery. The technique is described as *percutaneal transluminal coronary angioplasty* (*PTCA*). It is primarily used to treat patients with disabling angina who might otherwise be candidates for bypass surgery.

The procedure is performed as follows: a relatively large catheter, called a guiding catheter, is introduced percutaneously through either a femoral or a brachial artery and positioned at the ostium of the involved vessel. Coronary angiography is performed through the guiding catheter to visualize the exact location of the lesion. A second catheter – the coronary dilation catheter – is then inserted through the guiding catheter to the site of obstruction. The dilatation catheter, which has a short, flexible wire guide at its tip, is advanced until the guide wire passes through the obstruction and the deflated balloon section of the catheter straddles the stenotic area (Fig. 3.2). The balloon is then inflated for 3–5 seconds with a pressure sufficient to dilate the obstructed segment. If the first response is not satisfactory, the inflation cycle may be repeated several times. After the procedure, patients are monitored for 6–8 hours and may be discharged after 1–2 days. [The problems and counterindications are described and a measured statement concludes the section.] Further evaluation of the benefits, risks, and long-term effects of PTCA will be necessary to define the eventual role of this innovative method of treatment.

(Meltzer, Pineo and Kitchell 1983 p. 28, figure on p. 29)

Catheterisation: a novel view

'They're dying to cut into me and do a bypass. But there's this less radical option they can do first and l am supposed to see a guy up here at St Joseph's about having it done this spring. It's called an angioplasty. There's a balloon on the end of a catheter a yard long at least. They thread up into your heart from a cut they make just under your groin, the artery there. I had it done kind of in Florida but instead of a balloon it was a bunch of dyes they put in to see what my poor old ticker actually looked like. It's a funny experience: it doesn't actually hurt but you feel very funny, demoralized like, while its being done and terrible for days afterward. When they put the dye in, your chest goes hot like you're in an oven. Deep, it feels too deep. Like having a baby but then no baby, just a lot of computerized bad news about your coronary arteries. Still it beats open heart where they saw through your sternum for starters' – He touches the center of his chest and thinks of Thelma's breasts . . . 'and then run all your blood through a machine for hours. I mean, that machine is you for the time being. It stops, you die.'

(Updike 1990 p. 164)

Myocardial infarction: a nursing text

Most patients with acute myocardial pain seek medical assistance because of *chest pain*. The pain is usually quite distinctive; it occurs suddenly and is of severe, crushing quality. It is more intense than the pain of angina or the intermediate coronary syndrome and may be unlike any sensation the patient has experienced previously. Typically, the pain is concentrated directly beneath the sternum, but it frequently radiates across the chest or to the arms and neck. Patients commonly describe the pain as a heavy weight or pressure or knot in the chest. Unlike angina, the pain does not necessary occur with exertion; in fact, it frequently begins during sleep. Its occurrence after eating explains why many patients interpret the pain as indigestion. The chest pain is continuous and is not relieved by change in body position, breath holding, or by home remedies (e.g. bicarbonate) the patient may try. It usually persists for 30 minutes or more and may not subside until morphine is administered. Nitroglycerin seldom influences the duration or severity of the pain, shortly after the onset of the substernal pain drenching perspiration usually begins, and nausea and vomiting often occur at the same time, fear and apprehension are usual and most patients sense that a catastrophe has happened.
Meltzer, Pineo and Kitchell 1983 p. 13)

Myocardial infarction: a novel view – Updike (through Rabbit and Charlie) poses the dialectic of somatic and incarnate

'Sure, easy for you to say. People die having these things. I notice you never had one.'

'But I did. In '87. December, you were in Florida. They replaced two valves. Aortic and mitral. When you have rheumatic fever as a kid, it's the valves that go. They don't close right. That's what gives you the heart murmur, blood running the wrong way.'

Rabbit can hardly bear these images, all these details inside him, valves and slippages and crusts on the pipe. 'What'd they replace them with?'

'Pig heart valves. The choice is that or a mechanical valve, a trap with a ball. With the mechanical you click all the time. I didn't want to click if I could help it. They say it keeps you awake.'

'Pig valves.' Rabbit tries to hide his revulsion. 'Was it terrible? They split your chest open and ran your blood through a machine?'

'Piece of cake. You're knocked out cold. What's wrong with running your blood through a machine? What else do you think you are, champ?'

A God-made one-of-a kind with an immortal soul breathed in. A vehicle of grace. A battlefield of good and evil. An apprentice angel. All those things they tried to teach you in Sunday school, or really didn't try very hard to teach you, just let them drift in out of the pamphlets, back there in that church basement deeper in his mind than an air-raid shelter.

'You're just a soft machine,' Charlie maintains

(Updike 1990 p. 196)

Myocardial infarction: a novel view – the death of Rabbit

(Playing Basketball and (?) metaphorizing the life and death of White Middle Class, Middle America). Up he goes, way up towards the torn clouds. His torso is ripped by a terrific pain elbow to elbow. He bursts from within; he feels something immense persistently fumble at him, and falls unconscious to the dirt . . . Tiger . . . sees the big old white man, looking choked and kind of sleepy in the face, collapse soundlessly, like a rag doll being dropped.

'The infarction looks to be transmural,' Dr Olman tells Janice, and clarifies 'Right through the gosh-darn wall.' He tries to show her with the skin and flesh of his fist the difference between this and a sub-endocardial infarction that you can live with. 'Ma'am, the whole left ventricle is *shot*,' he says, 'my guess is there was a complete restenosis since this April's procedure up north.' His big face, with its sunburnt hooked nose and jutting Australian jaw, looks confusingly to Janice in her sleeplessness and grief like a heart itself. All this activity of the doctor's hands, as if he's trying to turn Harry inside out for her, now that it's too late. 'Too late for a bypass now,' Dr Olman almost snorts, and with an effort tames his voice into its acquired Southern softness. 'Even if by a miracle, ma'am, he were to pull through this present trauma, where you and I have healthy flexible muscle he'd just have a wad of scar tissue. You can replace arteries and valves but there's no substitute yet for live heart muscle.' He exudes controlled anger, like a golfer who has missed three short putts in a row. He is so young Janice groggily thinks, he blames people for dying. He thinks they do it to make his job more difficult.

(Updike 1990 pp. 420–1)

Post-Script

Angina: a nursing text (signs, discontinuities, analyses)

Angina: a medical text (historical, comprehensive, contextualised, cautiously definitive but magisterial)

Angina: a novel view (feelings, continuities, syntheses) Updike (through Rabbit and Charlie) poses the dialectic of somatic and incarnate

I do not want at this point to offer readers a definitive set of lessons I have taught, or conclusions which I feel that they must draw, hence ephemeral Script rather than fixed Text or the mere unsituated Word with which I began. Looking at the texts which I have presented and taking angina as the example, I have signalled the existence of a continuum. This starts from a view of the body as an object in the discourses embedded in the medical text to the patients' view of themselves as living subjects. I have suggested that the former is both made possible by a partly beneficial view of the body as mechanism, situated in the enduring history of 'Cartesian' Western world views, but expounded in the medical texts as a history of individual discoveries. These are seen as cumulative leading to a professionally scientific correction of errors (although Descartes, unlike many of his successors, was well aware of the limitations of the machine as model and reality (see Lawler 1991 pp. 55–6; Dreyfus 1992).

The medical text cited is a document of a frontier which is already established. This is signified by the magisterial authority and titled majesty of its progenitor. The story of angina's past, however, is presented in order that it remains clear that its history may continue and understanding be even more precisely refined. The text is an invitation to neophytes to master but also perhaps to transcend. The clinical problem of angina is defined (i.e. its limits set) by being given both boundary and context. Students have potential planning permission to extend or interfill the edifice. They are not, however, expected to need or want to demolish and rebuild.

The specific nursing text I have used translates the medical text in very precisely limited ways. It is a pragmatic manual for action based on need to know. It is an abstract, an almost diagrammatic mapping which knowingly reduces the riches and historical and contextual depth of its medical sources. The nurse is told enough to understand the doctors' concern to correct or mitigate the patients' disease. S/he is to be acquainted with the landmarks, the signs and symptoms but not with the systematic relationships between them. S/he does not need, in this view and within this discourse, to be given the knowledge to transcend them. The nursing text thus tolerates discontinuities; unattached parts of a system whose interrelations are not of necessity shown in their full interactions. For the doctor the disease's social relations are diachronically historical, situated in hospitals and laboratories, past and present. For the nurse the patient's synchronically social relations are in the ward and the operating theatre now and in the future. For the patient, harbouring and suffering the disease, and the disease itself are episodic and isolable in space and time.

This is not so of the patient's illness, as Updike's novel so brilliantly demonstrates. For each patient the disease *is* novel; an experience amongst experiences, a suffering among sufferings, a problem among problems all unique to him. It is cut off from the flow of life in neither space nor in time. What is uniquely cut off for patients is the experience of at once being in hospital and of being forced into a somatic view of their own bodies as against their more usual experience of selves incarnate.

As some recent radical nursing theorists and teachers have implied it is this difference between illness as flow and disease as episode which not only provides a source of alienation, for the suffering patient become an impatient sufferer, but which also provides the opportunity for nurses to transcend and encompass the medical model while retaining and employing to the full their clinical skills and experience. Gadow (1980), for example, in defining the nurse's role as existential advocacy, has suggested that the patient by being forced to focus on the physical body, either as a whole or in part, comes to experience what she calls the object body as separate from, and dominant over, the lived body. This may well be enhanced by its subjection to and replacement by technological devices as simple as intravenous drips or as complex as total life support machines. The nurse can help to restore the perception of the unity of object and lived body not only in the hospital where object dominates but in the world outside where the mutedness of the object body in relation to the lived may, as Marx notoriously but obliquely suggested in *The German Ideology* (1964 pp. 44–5), also present a form of alienation of species being. Oliver Sacks (1984) in a Jewish equivalent of the muscular Christian doctrine of *mens sana, in corpore sano* similarly presents the relationship of his corporeal and lived body as loss and restoration of unified control as he passes through the stages of injury, sufferer, patient, surgical intervention, postoperative patient, convalescence, rehabilitation and return to active life. (See Joy L. Johnson (1991) for a more schematised sociological application of this general idea to heart disease.)

Lawler (1990) following Gadow's philosophical arguments, has made the interaction on a holistic basis between the embodied selves of patients and their nurses the centre of her empirical study of what was happening on the wards of an Australian hospital and what ought to be the future of nursing. Benner (1984) has shown the consistency of these views of the nursing process with the way in which nurses move from 'novices to experts' in their craft. Anselm Strauss (1985) and his colleagues in their now classic studies of the various types of work process affecting the trajectory of sickness in the US hospital dominated by the high technology treatment of acute episodes of chronic disorder laid the foundations of the path followed here. What I hope I have begun to demonstrate through the juxtapositions of this chapter is that science-based technological medicine makes the central reality of patient experience of illness paradoxically even more relevant to healing than the person to person, 1/ thou, relationships of the theorists and chroniclers of traditional rural general practice (see for example Berger and Mohr 1976). Knowledge of this reality is not merely an adjunct to achieving compliance, as is illustrated in the discussion of explanatory models above. It offers a potential for the total subversion of the power structures of existing clinical practice which is already apparent to thinking nurses even if they lack the resources to put it into effect. It has yet to reach the textual conscience and consciousness of all medical and most patient-based discourse.

The three discourses described generate three types of expertise all of which appear to be essential to the most effective and life-enhancing use of technological opportunity. A set of concepts of the body which is at least partially shared may provide the new boundary object which makes mutual intelligibility possible after all.

REFERENCES

Armstrong, D. (1983), *Political Anatomy of the Body: Medical Knowledge in Britain in the Twentieth Century,* Cambridge University Press

Armstrong, D. (1985), 'Space and time in British general practice', *Social Science and Medicine,* xx, pp. 659–66

Bakhtin, M. (1984), *Rabelais and his World,* Indiana University Press, Bloomington

Benner, P. (1984), *From Novice to Expert: Excellence and Power in Clinical Nursing Practice,* Addison Wesley, Menlo Park, Calif.

Benner, P. and Wrubel, J. (1988), *The Problem of Caring,* Addison Wesley, Menlo Park, Calif.

Berger, J. and Mohr, J. (1976), *A Fortunate Man,* Penguin Books, Harmondsworth

Biale, D. (1985), 'Gershon Sholem's ten unhistorical aphorisms on Kabbalah: text and commentary', *Modern Judaism*, V, pp. 67–93

Bologh, R. (1979), *Dialectical Phenomenology: Marx's Method*, Routledge & Kegan Paul, London

—— (1981), 'Grounding the alienation of self and body: a critical phenomenological analysis of the patient in Western medicine', *Sociology of Health and Illness*, III, pp. 186–206

Bowker, G. and Star, L. S. (1990), 'Boundary objects, standards and long-term, large-scale co-ordination: the case of the international classification of diseases', Ms in author's collection

Comaroff, J. (1985), *Body of Power: Spirit of Resistance*, Chicago University Press

Dreyfus, H.L. (1992), *What Computers Still Can't Do: A Critique of Artificial Reason*, MIT Press, Cambridge, Mass.

Douglas, M. (1970 (1966)), *Purity and Danger*, Penguin Books, Harmondsworth

—— (1973), *Natural Symbols* (2nd edition), Barrie & Jenkins, London

Farmer, P. (1988), 'Bad blood, spoiled milk: bodily fluids as moral barometers in rural Haiti', *American Ethnologist*, XV, pp. 62–83

—— (1990), 'Sending sickness: sorcery, politics, and changing concepts of AIDS in rural Haiti', *Medical Anthropology Quarterly* (NS) IV, pp. 6–27

—— (1992), *AIDS and Accusation: Haiti and the Geography of Blame*, University of California Press, Berkeley

Gadow, S. (1980), 'Existential advocacy: philosophical foundation of nursing', in S. F. Spicker, S. Gadow, (eds.) *Nursing: Images and Ideals, Opening Dialogue with the Humanities*, Springer Publishing Co. New York

Handelman, S. A. (1991), *Fragments of Redemption*, Indiana University Press, Bloomington

Hill, P. (1992), *A Good Death*, Merloyd Lawrence Books, Addison Wesley, New York

Jacobs, J. (1988), *Doctors and Rules: A Sociology of Professional Values*, Routledge, London

Johnson, J. L. (1991), 'Learning to live again: the process of adjustment following a heart attack', in J. M. Morse, and J. L. Johnson (eds.), *The Illness Experience: Dimensions of Suffering*, Sage, London, pp. 13- 88

King, J. L. and Star, S. L. (1990), 'Conceptual foundations for the development of organizational decision support systems', Conference paper, Hawaian International Conference on Systems Science, January

Kleinman, A. (1980), *Patients and Healers in the Context of Culture*, University of California Press, Berkeley

—— (1988), *The Illness Narratives: Suffering, Healing and the Human Condition*, Basic Books, New York

Laqueur, T. (1990), *Making Sex: Body and Gender from the Greeks to Freud*, Harvard University Press, Cambridge, Mass.

Lawler, J. (1991), *Behind the Screens: Nursing Somology and the Problem of the Body*, Churchill Livingstone, Edinburgh

Lecercle, J.-J. (1990), *The Violence of Language*, Routledge, London

Marx, K. (1951 (1897)) *The 18th Brumaire of Louis Bonaparte . . . The Story of a Sawdust Caesar*, tr. Daniel De Leon, Labor News Company, New York

Marx, K. and Engels, F. (1965 (1844–6)), *The German Ideology*, Lawrence and Wishart, London

Mauss, M. (1973 (1935)), *Techniques of the Body*, tr. Ben Brewster, in *Economy and Society*, II, pp. 70–88

MacLeod, R. and Lewis, M. (eds.), (1988), *Disease. Medicine and Empire*, Routledge, London

Meltzer, L. E., MD , Pinneo, R., RN, MS and Kitchell, J. R., MD (1983), *Intensive Coronary Care: A Manual for Nurses*, 4th edition, Prentice-Hall International Editions, Englewood Cliffs, N.J.

Monks, J. and Frankenberg R. (1994), 'Being ill and being me: self, body and time in MS narratives' in B. Ingstad and S. Reynolds Whyte (eds.) *Culture and Disability*, University of California Press, Berkeley

Morse, J.M. and Johnson, J.L. (eds.) (1991), *The Illness Experience: Dimensions of Suffering*, Sage, London

Ots, T. (1990), 'The angry liver, the anxious heart and the melancholy spleen: the phenomenology of perceptions in Chinese culture, *Culture, Medicine and Psychiatry*, XIV, pp. 21–58

Radley, A. (1988), *Prospects of Heart Surgery: Psychological Adjustment to Coronary Bypass Grafting*, Springer Verlag, New York

Romanyshin, R.D. (1989), *Technology as Symptom and Dream*, Routledge, London

Sacks, O. (1984), *No Leg to Stand On*, Picador, London

Scheper-Hughes, N. and Lock, M. (1987), 'The mindful body: a prolegomenon to future work in medical anthropology', *Medical Anthropology Quarterly NS* I, pp. 16–41

Scott, Sir R. B., KCVO, MA, DM, FRCP, Physician to HM The Queen (ed.) (1973), *Price's Textbook of the Practice of Medicine*, 11th edition, Oxford University Press

Shepherd, M. P. (1990), *Heart of Harefield: the Story of the Hospital*, Quiller Press, London

Spicker, S. F. and Gadow, S. (eds.) (1980), *Nursing: Images and Ideals. Opening Dialogue with the Humanities*, Springer Publishing Company, New York

Stafford, B.M. (1991), *Body Criticism: Imaging the Unseen in Enlightenment Art and Medicine*, MIT Press, Cambridge, Mass.

Star, S.L. (1988), 'The structure of ill-structured solutions: boundary objects and heterogeneous distributed problem solving', in L. Gasser, and M. Huhns, (eds.), *Distributed Artificial Intelligence* 2, Morgan Kauffman, Menlo Park, Calif.

Star, S. L. and J. R. Grisemer, (1989), 'Institutional ecology, translations and boundary objects: amateurs and professionals in Berkeley's Museum of Vertebrate Zoology, 1907–1939', *Social Studies of Science*, XIX, pp. 387–420

Stimson, G. and Webb, B. (1975), *Going to See the Doctor: The Consultation Process in General Practice*, Routledge & Kegan Paul, London

Strauss, A., Fagerhaugh, S., Suczek, B., and Wiener, C. (1985), *Social Organization of Medical Work*, University of Chicago Press

Taussig, M. (1992), 'Reification and the consciousness of the patient', in *The Nervous System*, Routledge, New York and London, Chapter 6

Updike, J. (1990), *Rabbit at Rest*, Fawcett Press, New York

Vaughan, M. (1991), *Curing Their Ills: Colonial Power and African Illness*, Polity, Cambridge

Winterson, J. (1992), 'The cells, tissues, systems and cavities of the body', *The Body*, Granta, XXXIX (spring), pp. 126–36

Wolf, Z. R. (1988), *Nurses' Work. The Sacred and the Profane*, University of Pennsylvania Press, Pa.

PART FOUR

Understanding the social role and development of high technology medicine

13

Lay perceptions of modern medicine and medical practice

MICHAEL CALNAN AND SIMON WILLIAMS

INTRODUCTION

The public's beliefs and feelings as a whole about modern medicine appear to be a much neglected issue. Studies of patient satisfaction with patient care have tended to show that patients are rarely critical of medical practice (Calnan 1984, 1988a). This is in many respects surprising, given that some studies have highlighted the constant possibility of strain and tension in the doctor-patient relationship because of the many ways in which such encounters can prove unsatisfactory. One possible source of strain is that medicine cannot successfully solve all the problems with which it is presented. Yet, where criticisms are found, they usually focus on the *personal* qualities of the doctor or on his or her performance within the consultation, such as the ability to listen to patients' stories, to reassure them, or to clearly communicate information about the patients' complaints (Williams and Calnan 1991). Patients rarely tend to be critical of the actual modern medicine, or medical technology which they consume, at least according to this evidence.

This lack of patient criticism of medical practice and, to a greater extent of modern medicine itself, might reflect a 'managerial bias' in the studies which have been conducted, or the dominance of certain methodological approaches (Calnan 1988a). Alternatively, it may validly reflect a high level of public satisfaction or a lack of concern about medicine and medical matters.

Some sociologists working at the macro level (Parsons 1951; Illich 1975; Waitzkin 1979) have tended to agree with the former explanation. They have made the assumption that the public accepts that modern medicine is effective and thus has complete faith in the value of scientific medical knowledge. Similarly, social historians (Larson 1978), tracing the development of modern medicine and the rise of the medical profession, have suggested that during the course of the nineteenth century the public's views about scientific medicine were changed from suspicion to a general acceptance. Others, however, have been less concerned with the public's perceptions, as their theories suggest that power lies in the control over knowledge, and the practices and structures which sustain it. For example, Foucault (1973) suggests that the ways in which we perceive and speak about the body and medical matters is the product of the wider historical conditions and power relations within society which shapes and conditions both knowledge base, and hence the prevailing mode of discourse of the world in which we live.

Thus, for Foucault, the body is a product of a subtle play of power which is constituted by the clinical gaze. The implication is that the congruence between the prevailing dominant medical discourse and lay perceptions is not a relevant issue as lay perceptions have limited influence. As Turner (1984) points out, this 'discourse determinism' leaves little room for subjectivity and embodiment and thus fails to provide an adequate phenomenology of the body. For example, Turner emphasises the importance of human agency and consciousness and this is expressed un the language of ownership used in relation to the body.

The theoretical issue, however, of the potential for differences between levels of discourse appears to have been addressed directly by Cornwell (1984) in her ethnographic study of lay accounts of health and illness. Cornwell draws on the work of Habermas (1971) who makes a distinction between what she terms 'traditional legitimations', which are concerned with issues of human value which are tied to religious, philosophical and moral belief systems; and modern legitimations, which are scientific and technical and are founded upon empirical and analytical knowledge.

The process of 'rationalisation' occurs as social life is transformed as traditional legitimations are replaced by modern legitimations. Moreover, this process occurs at two different levels; at the level of culture as a whole – what Habermas (1971) terms 'rationalisation from above' – and at the individual and/or sub-cultural level (i.e. 'rationalisation from below'). As Cornwell (1984) notes, medicalisation 'from above' concerns the changes in the Western view of mind and body which have occurred as a result of scientific medicine. In contrast, medicalisation 'from below' relates to the changes in both social life and individuals, and sub-cultural groups to accept these modern legitimations for health and illness *vis-à-vis* thetraditional (commonsense and moralistic) legitimations which have hitherto held sway within the lay populace. It also relates to the impact which the practical achievements of modern scientific medicine make on the 'collective consciousness'.

As Cornwell goes on to note, the advantage of using this conceptual framework for understanding the process of medicalisation:

> lies in the acknowledgement that the relationships of lay people to medicine, and thus by extension, to matters of health and illness more generally, can be analysed on different levels. It states the dominant tendency in our culture, which is towards modern scientific and techni- cal forms of legitimation, without implying that the process will neces- sarily be carried through everywhere and in all social groups, at the same pace or at the same time. The rate of progress of medicalisation depends upon the state of readiness of the sub- cultures and individuals within sub-cultures to allow it to take place, and on their state of awareness and knowledge of scientific achievements.
>
> (1984, p. 120)

Some of these examples illustrate the range of theoretical perspectives which have attempted to explain the link between the micro and macro levels. There has also been a similar range of perspectives to explain the role and impact of another crucial element, namely the role and impact of the mass media. For example, when examining the role which the media performs prevailing models suggest that it may have one of three functions. These are as follows: the mass manipulation of public opinion (the 'duped' model); the education of public opinion by independent professional journalists (the 'enlightenment' or 'demystification' model), or finally, responding to the demands of the lay populace for 'newsworthy' stories (the 'consumerist' model) (Manning 1985).

This leads us to another issue which is perhaps of more direct relevance to the question examined in this chapter, namely the influ- ence of the mass media upon lay thinking. The logic of the models outlined above would seem to suggest a different relationship between the public and the media. The mass manipulation and to some extent the education model assume a passive acceptance of infor- mation, whereas others suggest a more active role for public. Further- more, Hall (1981) also sees that the public is not necessarily duped by the media due to what he terms the 'encoding/decoding' process whereby media messages are encoded in a particular form but may be decoded by the lay populace in a variety of ways, ones which may not necessarily be those intended by the media.

The aim of this study is to shed some light on the value of these particular theoretical approaches through examining lay perceptions of modern medicine and medical practice. It builds on previous exploratory work (Calnan 1988; Gabe and Calnan 1989) which show that while there was considerable faith in modern medicine, technology was seen in a far more critical light. Certainly, the greatest criticisms focused on the use of drugs, whereas procedures such as heart transplants were believed to be making an important contribution. However, this research was restricted, not least because it only focused on women's perceptions. The aim of this chapter is to further examine these issues by drawing upon both quantitative survey data and in-depth qualitative interviews, which compare both men and women as well as covering a wider age range. The analysis breaks down and separates out different aspects of medical practice to see if and why people favour or are sceptical about specific technological procedures.

Following Banta (1983), we take medical technology to mean 'the drugs, devices, and medical and surgical procedures used in medical care and the organizational and support systems within which such care is provided'. The aim of selection was to attempt to span the broad spectrum of contrasting medical interventions which ranged from those of a more common everyday nature, such as antibiotics; those of a high technology life saving nature, such as heart transplants, and those areas of more recent technological innovation such as test-tube babies. For example, do the people who approve of transplants feel the same way about operations such as hysterectomies? Also, are so- called anti-drug feelings widespread, or are they specific to groups that are more likely to have drugs prescribed for them?

METHODS AND DATA FOR THE STUDY

The data, were drawn principally, from two sources. One of these was a survey carried out in 1988 on a random sample of the population in a local health district in Kent, England, who were aged 18 and over. Data were collected through self-completed questionnaires on general issues associated with satisfaction with health care and included a set of questions about the extent to which respondents would accept the doctors recommendation for: (1) the prescription of antibiotics; (2) a hernia operation; (3) an operation for bowel cancer; (4) the prescription of tranquillisers; (5) a hip replacement operation; and finally (6) a hysterectomy. In addition, a general question was asked about the extent to which the respondent had a general faith in doctors. As the questions asked related to the acceptance of medical advice to have these various procedures, it was decided that respondents should only reply to the questions which were *directly* applicable to them. Thus women were not asked about their acceptance of vasectomy and likewise, men were not asked about their acceptance of hysterectomy.

The questions were completed by 62 per cent (454) of the original sample of 735. Although of course no information is available concerning the characteristics of non-respondents there appears to be no obvious indications that the sample is systematically biased in any way. For example a comparison between the age and sex composition of our sample and the Canterbury and Thanet adult population in Kent shows little difference. In our study 45 per cent were male and 55 per cent were female compared with 47 per cent and 53 per cent respectively in the Canterbury and Thanet adult population as a whole for 1988. Similarly there was little difference between the age composition. For example, using the age bands (18–44), (45–64) and (65 plus) for comparative purposes, the respective percentages in our sample compared to the Canterbury and Thanet adult population as a whole were as follows: 41 per cent compared to 49 per cent (18–44 age group); 31 per cent compared to 26 per cent (45–64 age group), and finally; 28 per cent compared to 25 per cent (65 plus age group).

Regarding the statistical analysis of the data, the main procedures used were those of cross tabulation – using the Chi square test as a measure of statistical significance. Concerning the quantitative survey data, only associations and relationships which were statistically significant at the $p < 0.05$ level are reported.

The second source of data was collected from qualitative interviews with both partners where couples were married or living as married. The households were divided into ten couples from professional backgrounds and ten from manual backgrounds. The male partner was aged between 40 and 60. Similar medical procedures were examined and these included respondents' perceptions of the relative strength and weakness of the following: (1) antibiotics; (2) heart transplants; (3) test-tube babies; (4) hip replacements; (5) tranquillisers; (6) vasectomy; (7) hysterectomy; and finally (8) hernia. Also, questions were asked about their general faith in modern medicine. The two groups were selected from a representative sample of the Canterbury and Thanet population who had already taken part in a recent health promotion survey. This sampling frame enabled the two groups to be identified by social class, age, marital status and educational background although not by housing tenure and ethnic group. Thus, all men 40 to 55 who were married or living as married were identified. These were then divided into those from social classes one and two and those from social classes four and five. In an attempt to allow for educational background, only men reported leaving full time education at 17 or at a later age were included in the middle-class group and only men who left school at 15 or earlier were included for selection in a working-class group. The sampling frame identified 19 potential middle-class contacts of which ten couples were successfully interviewed. In the working-class group, 21 possible contacts were identified and ten couples were successfully interviewed. The interviews were carried out during 1988 and 1989 in the homes of the respondents by a female interviewer. On average there was a two week interval between the interview with the man and the interview with his partner. A similar schedule was used for both males and females. The questions on scientific medicine came at the end of the two hour interview.

The two studies generally had different aims, the survey was concerned with consumer satisfaction with health care (Williams and Calnan 1991), the qualitative study was concerned with a range of issues such explaining the relationship between social position, the salience of health and health related behaviour (Calnan and Williams 1991); thus questions about lay evaluations of health care and medical technology were of relevance to both these studies. In a previous paper (Calnan 1988a) it has been suggested that this topic is most fruitfully explored through qualitative methods, however, the relative neglect of the question suggests the need for collection of survey data in order to identify broader patterns and trends within the lay population.

Thus, whilst the quantitative data provide information concerning basic frequencies of response and of statistical relationships between the data, the exact meaning and interpretation of such data remains problematic. Hence the aim of including the data from the qualitative study, was in order to flesh out in more substantive detail the meaning of the findings established within the quantitative survey. We do of course recognise that the data collected via these differing methodologies, and the contexts within which they were elicited, may or may not necessarily yield complementary results. However, implicit in our approach concerning this particular topic, we view the methodologies adopted as stemming from a broadly similar positivistic paradigm which incorporates the issue of meaning (Brown and Harris 1978; Silverman 1985).

A good illustration of these issues, concerns the interpretation of 'ambivalence' in respondents' accounts. Clearly the nature of the responses generated within the survey data may yield apparently 'ambivalent' feelings towards certain specific forms of modern technology, yet the precise meaning of this 'ambivalence' remains unclear. In contrast, the qualitative data allows for the expression of a far more subtle and detailed account of ambivalent feelings regarding these particular issues; one which enables the juxtaposition of an number of thoughts and reflections upon the specific issue under consideration.

In presenting our quantitative and qualitative findings, it was decided that the most fruitful method was to look at them together, procedure by procedure. Hence it is to a discussion of each of the above procedures, at both a quantitative and qualitative level, that the paper now turns. The basic findings regarding the quantitative study are given in Table 13.1.

Medicines and Drugs

Antibiotics

The quantitative analysis showed that antibiotics were widely accepted by the respondents as being of value. For example 95 per cent of the sample said that they would accept the doctor's prescription of antibiotics. The quantitative analysis which looked at beliefs about antibiotics by gender, age, education, social class and health status showed that the only statistically significant difference concerned social class. That is to say, the working class were far more likely to accept antibiotics without question.

A similar pattern emerged from the qualitative analysis in that the majority of respondents expressed positive opinions with respect to antibiotics. However, there was nonetheless a frequently expressed caveat: namely, that antibiotics were alright provided they were not 'abused' or 'over-prescribed' as, due to the risk of immunity, their efficacy would decline. This issue appeared to be more often raised by women rather than men (13 vs 7), and middle-class respondents

Table 13.1 Summary of basic findings regarding the lay evaluation of modern
medical technology

Doctor's recommendation	Accept without question	Accept with explanation	Not readily Not at all
Antibiotics			
%	54	41	5
N	(239)	(180)	(20)
Hernia operation			
%	30	63	7
N	(118)	(251)	(27)
Bowel cancer operation			
%	29	60	12
N	(119)	(249)	(48)
Tranquillisers			
%	8	29	63
N	(35)	(120)	(262)
Hip replacement			
%	25	62	13
N	(100)	(243)	(51)
Hysterectomy			
%	20	65	16
N	(43)	(138)	(32)
Faith in doctors	Lot of faith	Quite a lot	Not very much
%	31	56	13
N	(133)	(243)	(56)

Note: Numbers may not total 454 for each question due to the exclusion of those who did not
answer or for whom the question was N/A.

rather than working-class respondents (13 vs 7). For example, this
was a response from a middle-class woman:

'Well I mean antibiotics have revolutionised treatment haven't they?'
'In what way?'
'Well because people just died by the score didn't they, but antibiotics
now enable people to recover.'

The question of 'over-usage' or 'abuse' was again well illustrated by a
middle-class woman:

'If they are not abused and used in moderation, yes ... We've got a
great problem if they are abused because that means that we have got
to go on and develop different types of antibiotics, because the more

frequent penicillins have been abused and bacteria have become immune to them.'

In general, therefore, antibiotics were seen to be beneficial when used in moderation.

Tranquillisers

Although anti-drug feelings did not manifest themselves with respect to antibiotics the reverse was true for tranquillisers. Of the sample, 33 per cent said that they would not readily accept doctors' recommendations for tranquillisers and another 30 per cent said that they would reject the doctor's recommendation altogether. Age, gender, social class, educational and health status, all appeared to be associated with beliefs about tranquillisers. Thus those who were younger, were women, were from middle-class backgrounds, were more highly educated and whose health status was perceived as 'good', all appeared more critical of tranquillisers.

These negative or ambivalent feelings about the prescription and usage of tranquillisers were well illustrated by the qualitative data. None of the study group were wholly positive in their evaluation of tranquillisers. There also appeared to be some social-class variations in that working-class respondents tended to express negative/critical attitudes, whereas middle-class respondents tended to express more ambivalent attitudes (13 vs 3 critical, and 7 vs 19 ambivalent). There were four respondents amongst the working-class respondents (all women) who reported previous use of tranquillisers compared with only one man and one woman in the middle-class group.

There were three main reasons why negative comments were expressed. First, that they were or could be 'addictive'. For example, a working-class response:

> 'No I don't believe in tranquillisers, not really . . . Well they can get a hook on you and trying to get off them is very, very hard, if you can do without, I would say yes, do without.'

The second reason was that they were given too frequently. As a working-class woman stated:

> 'They are addictive, I don't care what you say, and if it keeps the patient quiet, then I think the doctors issue them willy-nilly. I mean, when I was having problems with Andrew, doctor W said to me "You know, I can put you on tranquillisers." But I said "Oh no, I couldn't have that." Well they don't make the problems go away, they just dull them don't they.'

This last quotation also illustrates the third explanation, in that tranquillisers made the problem more tolerable but didn't really deal with the root cause.

The ambivalent attitudes mainly expressed by the middle-class respondents also recognised these negative elements, but also tended to stress that they did have a place or function in certain specific cases – such as short-term management crises – if used prudently and monitored closely. For example a middle-class woman said about tranquillisers:

> 'Only in extreme cases. I don't think they solve the problem that is causing the need for them.You have got to get to the bottom of the problem. I don't think they are a good idea, only in extreme cases. Maybe you have a bereavement and something drastic has happened to you and you need a little help for a little while, well maybe it's OK, but not the way they are dished out year-after-year.'

Hence the overwhelming impression gained from the data regarding tranquillisers was of criticism and/or rejection. This could be contrasted with the beliefs about antibiotics. Certainly, there was evidence of an anti-tranquilliser culture amongst the lay population.

Elective surgery

Hip replacement
At a general level, the majority of people appeared to whole heartedly endorse the benefits of hip replacement. For example 25 per cent said that they would accept the doctor's recommendation without question and another 60 per cent said that they would accept it with explanation. However, there were interesting differences in response according to age, gender and educational status. Older people (60 plus) were more likely than their younger counterparts to accept the doctor's recommendation without question, and this was also the case for men compared with women and those who left school at 16 years of age or less.

The popularity of hip replacements was also clearly evident in the qualitative data. The benefits they bestow in terms of a reduction in pain and suffering and improved quality of life were extolled by the vast majority of respondents irrespective of class or gender. For example, this was illustrated from the comment from a working-class man:

> 'Yes, great . . . Well my mother-in-law, for instance, she's had two done,

and seeing the pain and the agony she was in before, I think they are doing absolute wonders for the patients who need them. Yes, I think it's wonderful.'

And, from a middle-class man:

'I think they are a very important operation. A lot of patients have had a second lease of life from the operation.'

The one note of dissent, came from a middle-class man:

'I have not know personally anybody who has had a completely success-ful hip operation, they really don't seem to be that comfortable after-wards. No I don't think . . .'

Thus it seemed that this particular form of medical technology was one of the most highly regarded and praised form of intervention, possibly because its benefits were so readily apparent in terms of reducing pain and suffering, increasing mobility and improving the quality of life of those who had them.

Hernia operations
As with hip replacements, hernia operations were also a form of medical technology which received widespread support. For example, 30 per cent accepted the doctor's recommendation without question and 63 per cent said that they would accept it with an explanation. Beliefs about hernia operations varied by age and class. That is to say, younger and middle-aged people were much less likely to accept a hernia operation without question. This was also the case for people from working-class backgrounds.

The qualitative data also showed that hernia operations were uni-versally acclaimed by respondents within the study irrespective of class and gender. As with hip operations, it seemed that the benefits of hernia operations were readily apparent; mitigating pain and suffering and improving the quality of life. For example, a working-class man remarked:

'Well I look on that the same way as I do hip operations, without them I think we would be lost. Yes, I think the medical people and people who pioneered such operations, they have done a lot of good to mankind.'

Whilst a middle-class woman remarked:

'Oh yes, I think hernia operations for those who have the problem are very good and I wouldn't have thought they were tremendously expensive operations, and I think it is a great shame that very many people have to wait months on some occasions to have one done.'

Reproductive technology

Hysterectomy

Hysterectomy was also a popular operation. For example, 20 per cent of women said that they would accept the doctor's recommendation without question, and another 65 per cent said that they would accept the doctor's recommendation with an explanation. However, age, educational status and health status appeared to be associated with level of acceptance of the procedure. Thus those women who were younger, more highly educated and in 'good health', less readily accepted the doctors recommendations for a hysterectomy.

The qualitative data also showed that the benefits of hysterectomy were well accepted. For example, a working-class woman said:

'That's the womb being taken out isn't it? . . . If it's diseased. Yes, I believe in having it taken away.'

And a middle-class woman stated:

'I would say, yes, because I've got so many friends who have had them and are living such a much better quality of life, so I would say yes.'

In contrast to this majority viewpoint, two middle-class women expressed certain qualifications about the wholesale endorsement of this procedure. For example, one middle-class woman said:

'If it's really, really necessary. A lot of it is only son of hearsay, you know, people have hysterectomies who really can't be bothered with the change, you know, you hear these stories, and in certain cases, such as with cancer, you get no choice.'

Vasectomy

The issue of vasectomy was only explored through qualitative data. While there was little evidence of wholly negative beliefs about vasectomies, approximately equal numbers of working- and middle-class men were either positive or ambivalent regarding this procedure. For example, the following illustrate the positive comments given. First, a working-class man:

'Well, I think it's probably a good thing I suppose . . . Well I suppose it solves any unwanted babies or that sort of thing.'

Secondly, a middle-class man:

> 'Well, it's probably a good method of birth control. Recently, there has been some speculation that it does cause some health problems, but I don't really know that much about it.'

Next ambivalence, which often stressed that whilst respondents were not against vasectomies in principle, or which stressed the issue of choice, they themselves would not have it done as other less radical forms of birth control were available. For example, a middle-class man:

> 'They are sort of unnecessary really, unless it's essential. I don't know of any essential indications for a vasectomy.'

Whilst a working-class man remarked:

> Well I suppose they serve a purpose, I mean I'm not against birth control and things like that as such, but I mean there are other forms of birth control without vasectomy. I think it's a bit over-drastic.'

Test-tube babies

The final area of reproductive technology to be considered was that of test-tube babies. Once again, the analysis was based upon the qualitative data. This procedure generated a mixed response. Neither class, nor gender appeared to be systematically related to beliefs about this procedure. The sample was evenly split into two groups. First, there were those who were positively in favour, such as this working-class woman:

> 'Well, I think there are a lot of couples in the world who would like to have children but can't, so, yes, it's a help isn't it.'

Or, a middle-class woman in similar vein:

> 'Yes, yes, I think if a couple really long for a child, this is the only way they can do it, yes.'

However, the second group, were more ambivalent about this form of technology, and their ambivalence seemed to focus upon the fact that it was in some sense 'unnatural' or that it could be taken too far. For example, a middle-class woman said:

> 'There again, it's alright for me, I've got five. If I had got no children, then maybe I would go to any lengths to get a child and that would be quite acceptable. I think in moderation, but again it can be taken too far, genetics is a dodgy business.'

Or a working-class man:

> 'I don't altogether believe in that, I don't like it all. I think it should be a natural function between two parties, not done artificially in a test-tube.'

There was also another issue expressed, and that was the cost of such technology, *vis-à-vis* other competing needs and priorities. A final point was that in many of the respondents' accounts, there was a clear distinction between their general attitudes concerning the issue of test-tube babies and their opinions if their circumstances were different and they were childless.

In summary, in the three areas covered in this section on reproductive technology, there was evidence of a higher level of ambivalence expressed compared with the elective surgical procedures discussed in the previous section.

Life saving technology

The final form of technological intervention which was examined, focused upon procedures which related to life threatening diseases. The first of these, was heart transplants.

Heart Transplants

It was possible to divide the responses towards heart transplants into the following groups: the positive, and the ambivalent or critical. In this respect, middle-class respondents tended to be somewhat more ambivalent or critical than working-class respondents, and women generally more ambivalent or critical than men.

The positive responses were well illustrated in the following quotes. First from a middle-class man:

> 'Well, I think they can prolong someone's life, just for a few years possibly, and give them a better way of life for a short time, then they are a good thing.'

And a working-class woman:

> Yes, very good, it gives someone another lease of life, let's them live a bit longer, I'm all for that.'

It was possible to identify three main themes which underlay the replies of those who adopted a more ambivalent or critical stance. First, as with test-tube babies, there was a feeling that it was in some sense 'unnatural'. This is illustrated from the following two quotations, the first from a working-class man and the second from a working-class woman:

'Well I don't think that anybody should give transplants to other people because their heart is different from what the others' have been, it's unnatural isn't it.'

'Well I don't think you have a normal life afterwards . . . You have got to take drugs and the fear of rejection, that is kept very, very quiet I think, and I think it is still in the experimental stage at the moment.'

The second theme was associated with the religious, ethical and moral dilemmas involved. For example, a working-class woman remarked:

'I can't honestly say, probably if I needed one I'd be all for them. It's a very peculiar feeling I get, but I don't like the idea of them . . . I don't mind kidney transplants, but the heart . . . Perhaps it's sort of semi-religious, I really don't know, it's a bit sacrilegious.'

Or a working-class man:

I'm a bit unsure of this. I had one of those donor cards that you carry around. and I sat and looked at it and read it, and then I didn't sign it. It's a good thing, but there was a case on the radio today, Britain's youngest heart transplant, well it's alright providing it's going to be alright for her. But if it's kept her going for something else to go wrong and mess her up for the rest of her life, would they have been better leaving her as she was?'

The issue of age could also be included under this criteria. For example, a working-class woman stated:

'Not wishing to sound cruel, but I think heart transplants on younger people are more valuable than on older people . . . I feel that a man of 65 or over, who has had a good life, we accept that their time comes, but we don't accept that with a child of 19.'

Finally, the third theme to emerge from the accounts was that of economic cost and the management of finite resources within the health care field of competing needs and priorities. For example, one middle-class woman stated:

'If I had a husband who needed one, I'm sure I would be very positive, and I know that this is a very selfish attitude for me to take, but overall I think too much money is spent in this area and not enough in routine care.'

Of course, boundaries are never black and white, and the issue of resource allocation relates to the previous theme of moral and ethical dilemmas. Moreover. as with test-tube babies, another issue emerged, which was the conscious and open acknowledgment of a difference in attitude between, on the one hand, if the circumstances involved a loved one, and, on the other hand, their general attitudes and orientation towards this procedure.

Bowel cancer operations
In contrast to the previous area, the analysis of bowel cancer was based upon the quantitative data. The majority said that it would accept the doctor's recommendation to have an operation of this kind, with 29 per cent saying that they would accept it without question, and a further 60 per cent saying that they would accept the recommendation with an explanation. Older people (60 plus) appeared more accepting of the doctors recommendation for an operation for bowel cancer than did their younger counterparts.

In summary, of the two contrasting life saving operations considered here, heart transplants appeared to be more problematic in that they raised a number of fundamental moral and ethical issues concerning forms of modern technological intervention.

Faith in modern medical practice

Finally, more general questions were asked about respondents perceptions of their faith in modern medical practice.

Faith in doctors
Respondents in the survey were asked about their faith in doctors. Whilst 31 per cent expressed a lot of faith, 56 per cent expressed quite a lot of faith and 13 per cent not very much. These beliefs about doctors seemed to vary according to age, and educational status, and also according to health status over the last year. Older respondents, those who left school at 16 or before, and those who reported that their health in the last year had only been 'fair-poor', were significantly more likely to say that they had a lot of faith in doctors.

In addition, respondents' faith in doctors seemed be associated with some of the surgical procedures previously discussed, which were antibiotics, tranquillisers, hip replacements, hysterectomies, and operations for bowel cancer. Lack of faith in doctors appeared to be associated with scepticism about the value of each of these procedures.

Faith in modern medicine
As with the quantitative data analysis on faith in doctors, respondents generally seemed to have a considerable degree of faith in modern medicine as a whole. However, women tended to be slightly more ambivalent or critical than men. First, an example of the generally positive attitude displayed towards modern medicine. A working-class man:

> 'Yes, very good, I'm only going on what they have done for me wife over the last years, she had her valve done 15, 16 years ago.'

And a working-class woman:

> 'Well I think modern medical care now is much better because they can do a lot of things a lot better, and I think it will get better as it goes along.'

Secondly, there was the theme of ambivalent or criticism, particularly expressed by women. For example, a middle-class woman said:

> 'I think modern medicine is a two-edged weapon, I think because of the new drugs to help the diseases, it causes a lot of side-effects, and I am sure that now we have so many more medicines, we accordingly have a lot more disease caused by these medicines. I think it's a dual thing, I think it has got good and bad things.'

However, there was another quite different sort of ambivalence expressed towards modern medical care, one which did not criticise or question medicine *per se*, but rather criticised its organisation and funding. For example, a working-class man stated:

> 'Yes it could be a lot better if the money was forthcoming, if they were allowed to spend more and not keep having to close wards down, and hospitals even. It should be the other way round, they should be spending more on that.'

Whilst a middle-class man remarked:

> 'I have considerable faith in the ability of individuals in their field to treat, I have little faith in the NHS as such. I think the NHS tends to be unsatisfactory at the coal-face where it matters. I think it relies far too much on good-will and does not allow sufficient expertise to be applied.'

Thus, from the accounts presented, there appeared to be two levels at which the general question of faith in modern medicine as a whole was answered. At one level respondents answered in terms of faith and trust in modern medicine *per se*, and at the other level, respondents focused upon its current level of organisation and funding. However, the overall pattern which emerged at both levels, was on the whole positive.

A summary of the statistically significant relationships between the procedures considered above and certain basic socio-demographic data is given in Table 13.2.

Table 13.2 Summary of statistically significant relationships between acceptance of medical technology, socio-demographic and other health related variables

	Age	Gender	Education	Class	Health	Faith in doctors
Antibiotics				*		*
Hernia operation	*			*		
Bowel cancer	*					*
Tranquillisers	*	*	*	*	*	*
Hip replacement	*	*	*			*
Hysterectomy	*		*		*	*
Faith in doctors	*		*		*	

* χ^2 test: $p < 0.05$

DISCUSSION

In turning to a discussion of our findings, it seems that a number of points and issues emerge. First, our study supports the evidence from the previous exploratory study that the situation portrayed by some writers such as Illich (1975), of 'blanket dependence' or acceptance of modern medicine by the public is far too simplistic. Instead, as our findings have shown, views differ on the relative merits of modern medical technology according to which specific form of technological intervention is being considered (i.e. antibiotics, tranquillisers, hip operations, heart transplants etc.), and also in terms of the socio-demographic characteristics of the lay population (i.e. age, gender, class, educational status, health status etc.).

Indeed, our findings seem to suggest the following grounded typology of criteria utilised by the lay population when evaluating modern medical technology:

A typology of lay evaluative criteria
Outcome/evaluation

'Good'	'Bad'
Criterion/dimension	
Life saving	Life threatening
Quality of life enhancing	Quality of life diminishing
'Natural'	'Unnatural'
'Moral'	'Immoral'
'Necessary'	'Unnecessary'
Restoring independence	Promoting addiction/dependence
'Good value for money'	'Wast of money'

Thus, hip replacements, for example, tended to be regarded as 'good' due to their quality of life enhancing and independence restoring capacities. In contrast, tranquillisers tended to be seen as 'bad' as they were felt to be 'unnecessary', and also, more importantly, because they tended to lead to addiction and dependence. Again in contrast, test-tube babies tended to be predominantly evaluated in terms of the 'natural'/'moral' versus the 'unnatural '/'immoral' dichotomy; the outcome in many cases being one of expressed ambivalence. Similarly, concerning the issue of heart transplantation surgery, whilst many respondents concurred that it was life-saving and quality of life enhancing, the 'natural'/'un-natural' and the 'moral'/'immoral' dichotomies also tended to generate considerable ambiguity within the lay population about the benefits of this particular form of medical technology. Finally, particularly within the present economic and political context – one which increasingly stresses economic effectiveness, efficiency and value for money – there was also some evidence of a lay concern that due to the NHS's finite resources and the issue of competing priorities, certain forms of medical technology (e.g. heart transplants, test-tube babies) were too costly and that the money should instead be diverted elsewhere (e.g. to the care of the elderly) where the pay-off in terms of numbers treated would be greater.

Yet, at a theoretical level, what exactly does this tell us about the structure of lay thinking in relation to health care? Clearly, the medicalisation thesis has its explanatory limitations, particularly because it cannot account for the 'ambivalence' about modern scientific medicine expressed by the lay population. Do any of the other theoretical perspectives outlined earlier provide a more powerful explanation?

Cornwell's (1984) approach with its distinction between two levels of rationalisation is of value here. It is clear that rationalisation from below has indeed occurred, at least at the level of beliefs, its also clear that concerning certain specific forms of modern technological medicine, traditional beliefs and values hold greater sway. Thus, for example, whilst, hip replacements were wholeheartedly endorsed by the lay populace, tranquillisers, heart transplantation surgery and test tube babies seem to be in opposition to certain moral beliefs and values within the lay population.

There is evidence to suggest that these beliefs are at least in part a product of traditional values, in that work carried out on elderly populations (Calnan 1989) shows that, as with their younger counterparts, there was a strong anti-drug culture. These studies of elderly people have shown that while patients accepted doctors' prescriptions for medicines the patients never actually used their medications which were normally discarded. However, this may only provide a partial explanation in that rationalisation and medicalisation from above may also be under going a change. For example, twenty years ago the value of modern scientific medicine might have been less in doubt than it is now. Scientists are no longer the gods that they were twenty years ago and there is some evidence of disunity in the scientific community, although perhaps less so amongst the more tightly knit medical profession.

This demystification of science and scientific medicine may partly have been brought about due to the role of the mass media in society. and thus this may lend some support to the 'enlightenment' model outlined earlier. A good illustration of this concerns the media portrayal through 'atrocity tales' of tranquilliser dependence. However Gabe, Gustaffson and Bury (1991) suggest a slightly more subtle explanation for the influence of the media in the context of tranquilliser dependence. They suggest that the media actually performs more of a 'mediating' role between, on the one hand, the realm of individual experience and, on the other hand, media imperatives concerning the production of 'newsworthy' stories. Yet it must also be emphasised, as Karpf (1988) has pointed out, that the mass media may to a lesser extent be responsible for mystification, in that they may dramatise and amplify the success stories such as heart transplants and test tube babies. Thus, science and medicine have, to some extent, been demystified and the ambivalence expressed by respondents in these studies may reflect, at least in part, the impact of this demystification process.

The complexity of lay thinking can also be identified when the natural/unnatural dichotomy is turned to. It seems that certain specific forms of Western scientific medicine (e.g. test-tube babies) transgress or breach acceptable natural/unnatural boundaries maintained by the lay populace, ones which may vary by gender – i.e. what is 'natural' for men may be different to what is 'natural' for women – and represent an estrangement from nature and the natural course of life processes and production. Moreover, at another level, it may also be related to the traditional concern with, to quote an old adage, 'letting mother nature take its course', a 'return to nature', or to more 'natural' forms of therapeutic intervention. Consequently, in such circumstances, nature or the body is best left to 'its own devices' in order to heal itself naturally (i.e. via processes of homeostasis, balance and equilibrium) or instead, certain other forms of alternative medicine, ones which are 'loser to nature' such as homeopathy, are sought or turned to. Indeed, at a more theoretical level, Parsons (1978) makes a similar point when he introduces the notion of 'teleonymy'. This relates to the: 'healing power of nature . . . a property of living systems . . . by virtue of which such systems have a capacity to cope, often without outside intervention' (1978, p. 67, quoted in Gerhardt 1987, p. 119). As Gerhardt goes on to note, such teleonymy accounts for a vis medicatrix naturae; the implication being that the breakdown of teleonomic capacities (i.e. illness) *only* requires the *vis medicatrix* when nature fails to provide suitable and efficacious remedies (Gerhardt 1987).

Indeed, in the present context, the increasing number of the lay population who are turning to alternative/complementary forms of medicine and healing may perhaps symbolise an estrangement from, or a baulking against, contemporary forms of technological intervention which are felt in some way to be 'unnatural', coupled with a concern to return to more natural and hence to 'safer' forms of healing: a reflection of the increasing awareness of the limitations of scientific medicine.

A similar set of points can be made in relation to the issue of morality. In an increasingly secular world where 'science' and 'rationality' have to a large extent replaced religious and metaphysical systems of belief, there appears, at first sight, to be little room left for these more 'traditional legitimations' (Habermas 1971). As Turner (1987) notes, secularisation involves 'not only the decline of the Church, but also that the medical profession has replaced the traditional clergy as the group in society which manages normal relations' (1987, p. 219). Yet again, as our data suggest, the dispassionate rationality with which science and scientific advance is associated leads it into terrain and issues which clash rather than overturn certain fundamental religious, moral and ethical beliefs (Kennedy 1981). Consequently, ambivalent or critical attitudes are sometimes expressed towards certain forms of technological innovation concerned with issues of life and death. In this context, it is particularly interesting to note the ambivalence expressed towards heart transplants as being in a sense 'immoral', as the heart was a sacred object, the very core or essence of a person, and to remove it was in this respect sacrilegious.

Finally, at another level, the data also illustrates the differing sets of beliefs held by individuals according to whether the particular procedure(s) under consideration related to them or their family personally, or to members of the public in general. This may reflect the analytical distinction which Cornmwell (1984) draws between 'public' and 'private' accounts. In this particular context, public accounts may be characterised by a general ambivalence about various forms of modern technology whereas private accounts may be less concerned with wider issues of public principle and morality, and instead have a more self- interested focus. However, in this respect the content of public accounts may actually differ somewhat from that suggested by Cornwell, in that they may not simply reflect or reproduce dominant medical ideology but, instead, may stress traditional beliefs and ambivalence.

What of the nature of the social relations with modern medicine and is there any evidence to say that some social groups are more or less medicalised than others? For example, has womens' greater experience of health care led them to be more or less critical of scientific medicine? In a comparison between hysterectomy and vasectomy it would appear that women were more accepting of the former than men were of the latter. This may partly reflect the traditional gender division in responsibilities for contraception. Certainly, women seem to be more 'knowledgeable' than men which may reflect the different access to magazines, etc. No real equivalent of womens' magazines appears to be available for men. However, in relation to the other technological procedures considered, there was no evidence to say that women were any less critical than men; indeed, with respect to tranquillisers for example, they appeared more so. Thus, while the medicalisation theorists may be correct in asserting that women are more familiar with medical technology than their male counterparts, they are incorrect to assume that this necessarily leads to a less critical stance.

Unlike the previous research (Calnan 1988b) in which working-class women were more sceptical than their middle-class counterparts, the reverse was true in the studies presented in this chapter. Thus, the theories of Abercrombie and his colleagues (1988) may not be accurate in this context, as the criticisms by the middle class may be a product of the demystification process previously discussed.

Finally, as with other studies of lay evaluation and satisfaction there appears to be a positive relationship between age and acceptance and satisfaction with medicine. A number of explanations have been put forward for this and some of the most common imply either elderly people show greater deference or respect for medicine and doctors or they have low expectations of health and health care. Alternatively, with their greater general experience and the likelihood of their having more direct experience of the procedures themselves, elderly people may have a better understanding of the uncertainties and recognise that as medicine becomes more successful and expands its jurisdiction the more difficult the problems it will have to solve.

In conclusion this study has shown the limitations of the medicalisation thesis for explaining lay views about modern scientific medicine. The study shows that both men and women were ambivalent about the value of the number of available procedures and this was explained in part by reference to traditional values and the impact of the process of the demystification of modern medicine. Clearly the lay recourse to traditional values calls into question the Foucauldian 'discourse determinism' which Turner (1984) identifies. In this sense the emphasis upon unnatural aspects of modern medical technology may represent a symbolic struggle over control of the body.

REFERENCES

Abercrombie, N., Hill, S. and Turner, B.S. (1988), *The Dominant Ideology Thesis*, George Allen and Unwin, London

Banta, H. D. (1983), 'Social science research on medical technology: utility and limitations', *Social Science and Medicine*, XCII, pp. 1363–69

Brown, G. W. and Harris, T. O. (1978), *The Social Origins of Depression*, Tavistock, London

Bury, M. and Gabe, J. (1990), 'Hooked? Media responses to tranquilliser dependence', in P. Abbott and G. Payne, (eds.). *New Directions in the Sociology of Health (Explorations in Sociology No. 36)*, Falmer Press, Basingstoke, pp. 87–103

Calnan, M. (1984), 'Clinical uncertainty: is it a problem in the doctor-patient relationship?' *Sociology of Health and Illness*, VI, pp. 74–85

—— (1988a), 'Towards a conceptual framework for examining lay evaluation of health care', *Social Science and Medicine*, XXVII, pp. 927–38

—— (1988b), 'Lay evaluation of medicine', *International Journal of Health Services*, XVIII, pp. 311–22

Calnan, M. and Williams, S. J. (1991), 'Style of life and the salience of health: an exploratory study of health related practices in households from differing socio-economic circumstances', *Sociology of Health and Illness*, XIII, pp. 506–29

Calnan, S. E. (1989), 'Old people's perceptions of ageing and illness', unpublished MPhil. Thesis, Social Psychology, University of Kent

Cornwell, J. (1984), *Hard Earned Lives*, Tavistock, London

Foucault, M. (1973), *The Birth of the Clinic: An Archaeology of Medical Perceptions*, Tavistock, London

Gabe, J. and Calnan, M. (1989), 'The limits of medicine: women's perceptions of medical technology', *Social Science and Medicine*, XXVIII, pp. 223–31

Gabe, J., Gustaffson, U. and Bury, M. (1991), 'Mediating illness: media coverage of tranquilliser dependence', *Sociology of Health and Illness*, XIII, pp. 332–53

Gerhardt, U. (1987), 'Parsons, role theory and health interaction', in G. Scambler, (ed.), *Sociological Theory and Medical Sociology*, Tavistock, London, pp. 110–33

Habermas, J. (1971), *Towards a Rational Society*, Heinemann, London

Hall, S. (1981), 'Encoding/decoding television discourse', in S. Hall, *et al.* (eds.), *Culture Media and Language*, Hutchinson, London

Illich, I. (1975), *Medical Nemesis: The Expropriation of Health*, Care Calder and Boyar, London

Karpf, A. (1988), *Doctoring the Media*, Routledge, London

Kennedy, I. (1981), *The Unmasking of Medicine*, Allen and Unwin, London

Larson, M. (1978), *The Rise of Professionalism. A Sociological Analysis*, University of California Press, Los Angeles

Manning, N. (1985) (ed.), *Social Problems and Welfare Ideology*, Gower, London

Parsons, T. (1951), *The Social System*, Routledge and Kegan Paul, London

—— (1978), 'Health and disease: a sociological and action perspective', in T. Parsons, *Action Theory and the Human Condition*, Macmillan, London

Silverman, D. (1985), *Qualitative Methodology and Sociology*, Gower, Aldershot

Turner, B. (1984), *The Body and Society*, Blackwell, Oxford

—— (1987), *Medical Power and Social Knowledge*, Sage, London

Waitzkin, H. (1979), 'Medicine, superstructure and micro politics', *Social Science and Medicine*, III, pp. 601–19

Williams, S. J. and Calnan, M. (1991), 'Convergence and divergence: assessing criteria of consumer satisfaction across general practice, dental and hospital care settings', *Social Science and Medicine*, XXXIII, pp. 707–16

14

A social role for technology: making the body legible

DAVID ARMSTRONG

One of the earliest, if rudimentary, technologies deployed by modern medicine was the technique of percussion in which the density of the body's interior was explored by means of tapping chest and abdomen. There are records of its invention in the mid eighteenth century, but it was several decades before it came into general use. Contemporary religious sensibilities have been suggested as reasons for the delay in its application, in that it was not believed proper for the body to be examined in this way. Michel Foucault, however, in his seminal text on the birth of modern medicine, suggests that the reason for its delay was because the technology had no underlying theoretical model to justify its use (1973). Thus, eighteenth century humoral theories, which saw illness as moving throughout and outside of bodies, did not hypothesise that illness could be localised to one point and then be identified by spatial techniques.

The temporal separation of invention and application as found in the example of percussion supports the notion that the advent and growth of medical technology (particularly that of the clinical examination) is closely related to the model of illness which emerged in the closing decades of the eighteenth century, and which has since dominated Western thinking about health. Foucault characterised this novel framework for comprehending illness as the 'clinical gaze': he suggested this term to signify the centrality of a medical perception which sought to 'read' the human body. In other words the new medicine – which has since been called biomedicine or pathological medicine – came to see the human body as a text which could be made legible by techniques which penetrated its depths. Perhaps the classic example of such a technique was the invention of the stethoscope by Laennec in 1812. Put simply, the stethoscope extended the simple senses of the physician which were largely restricted to scanning the outside of the body, to enable its interior to become visible to the medical eye.

Contemporary advances in instrumentation, in techniques of the clinical examination, and in the all-important use of the post-mortem allowed physicians in the newly emergent neutral space of the hospital to explore, analyse, and thereby make legible the interior spaces of their patients' bodies in the constant search for the precise location of the pathological lesion. Yet Foucault also stressed that these new techniques did not represent enlightenment as is conventionally supposed, but rather a different way of reading the body. Foucault quotes Pomme, an eighteenth century physician, who treated a hysteric by making her take frequent baths and then reported seeing 'membranous tissues like pieces of damp parchment . . . peel away with some slight discomfort, and these were passed daily with the urine' and the intestines 'peeled off their internal tunics, which we saw emerge from the rectum' (1973 p. ix). To modern medical ears such claims are absurd, as are the old humoral theories of illness. There is an assumption that physicians in the eighteenth century and earlier could not have seen such phenomena, and consciously or unconsciously fooled themselves into believing that the manifestations of illness which they reported were visible. Foucault's response is to argue that this simply shows the incommensurability of different forms of perception: our modern way of seeing is unable to apprehend phenomena such as the humours just as the humoral physician was unable to perceive the analysable body constituted by tissues, cells and organs.

The great significance of the new medicine, however, did not lie simply in the technological advances which it used to make the body legible. In his later work, *Discipline and Punish: The Birth of the Prison* (1977) Foucault suggests that the parallel emergence in Western society of the hospital, the prison, the school, the barracks, and the workshop all represented the spread of techniques for making individuals' bodies legible – and hence the fabrication of the individual as a discrete entity. In Foucault's words these techniques brought 'ordinary individuality – the everyday individuality of everybody – [from] below the threshold of description' (1977 p. 191). In short, the various techniques of the early nineteenth century which played on the individual body and brought its anatomical structure into sharper focus were also techniques which in an important sense fabricated that very body as a social object. The early nineteenth century techniques which sought to make bodies legible also began to create individual bodies as they are perceived today. It is surely not coinciden-tal that the word individualism should originate at this time (Williams 1976), that it was discussed in political, economic and literary terms (Lukes 1973), and that, for the first time, individual bodies could be counted – witness the first national Census in Britain in 1801.

In summary, Foucault argued that a fundamental change occurred in Western society around the turn of the eighteenth century. A number of new techniques, rudimentary but pervasive, emerged to focus on the madman, the patient, the criminal, the school child, etc. Together these new techniques functioned to fabricate a discrete, passive, and analysable human body which could be transformed through these same techniques.

The priority given to making the body legible has continued for the last two centuries. Advances in instrumentation, in laboratory science, and in analytic techniques have enabled the investigation of the human body to operate at an increasingly detailed level, each time bringing into sharper focus the specific and reducible compo-nents which are believed to constitute the ultimate integrity of that body. Thus a large component of the history of medical technology can be explained as a continuation of this important social imperative to make the body legible. From haematology to clinical biochemistry, from radiology to biopsy, from surgery to pathology, there has been a great investment in the microanalysis of the human body over the last two centuries. Each of these developments has been construed as representing progress and advance because that is the vision behind the current Western conception of illness and the body. Ultimately, illness is reducible to a pathological lesion and the more the body can be made legible then the easier it will be to identify – and possibly remove – the localised basis of illness.

Of course, many illnesses defy such analytic procedures: psychiatric disorder and 'organic' symptoms without pathological correlates have continued to elude incorporation within this particular model of ill-ness. Nevertheless, the vision endures: ultimately technology will ensure that the visibility of the body is such that in the bright illumi-nation of the clinical gaze all illness – and the body that contains it – will be revealed to the penetrating eye of medicine. Of course, it is to be expected that every medical era will view its own perceptions as lying on the final road to full enlightenment. But there is evidence from earlier periods – with their similar claims to truth – that the current framework for understanding illness is neither the first nor the last. Thus, it might be expected, that other visions of illness, and new technologies to accompany them, will emerge in society; moreover, such changes may have already begun to occur and it is possible to discern a new, if inchoate, alternative model of illness which has emerged during the last few decades.

THE NEW SPACE OF ILLNESS

There is already a range of evidence available to support the emergence of a new model of illness (Armstrong 1983). Suffice it for this chapter to offer an illustration through the shifts in the medical gaze identifiable in the medical texts on clinical method published over the last few decades (Armstrong 1987). The fundamental techniques of making the body legible have been laid out for doctors in training in manuals of clinical method. During the early decades of the twentieth century these texts concentrated almost exclusively on the clinical examination to the exclusion of the patient's history: for example, Steven's *Medical Diagnosis* of 1910 offered only three pages out of 1500 to the 'interrogation of the patient'. At best the patient's words provided a somewhat unreliable pointer to the nature of the pathological lesion. Then, during the 1930s and 1940s, the new editions of these manuals began to add chapters on 'history-taking' – 'a subject to often omitted from books on diagnosis' (Cabot 1938). In part these new guides offered a more sophisticated analysis of how clinicians could get the pathology to speak 'through' the patient, but they also recognised that something else could intrude between the lesion and its visibility, and this was the idiosyncratic patient. Thus physicians were enjoined to ask their questions in certain ways to minimise the risk that patients might interfere with the purity of the lesion's manifestations in the form of symptoms.

Succeeding manuals began to develop further this new space of medical analysis. It was recognised, for example, that the patient's words not only represented the pathological lesion but also facets of the patient's emotional and social world. Thus, rather than solely exploring the space of the human body to make it reveal its secrets, medicine, over the last few decades has begun increasingly to explore the psychosocial world of the patient for its own inherent truths. In short, illness began to be transformed from what was visible to what was heard.

This shift in the medical interrogation can be summarised in the advice which was and is now offered to the neophyte physician: in the early nineteenth century the opening question was to take the form of 'Where is the pain?' or 'Where does it hurt?' or 'What is your complaint?' whereas nowadays it has been replaced by 'Now, please tell me your trouble' (McLeod 1976). In short, like the discovery of the body as an analytical space early in the nineteenth century, medicine has relatively recently discovered the psychosocial space of the patient as an analysable phenomenon. Clearly the techniques used to explore this space are not technological in the same sense as the machines which are used to explore anatomical space; and yet their purposes are parallel. Therefore, these techniques for making the psychosocial world of the patient legible can be seen as a new form of technology which is undergoing its own transformation and development, particularly under the guidance of psychologists, sociologists and those other 'human scientists' who increasingly infiltrate the world of medicine. Thus, it would appear that there are now two quite different 'gazes' interrogating the patient: on the one hand there is the physical technology which has offered a reductionist analysis of the anatomical body in its search for the pathological lesion, and on the other hand there are the new and developing techniques of the interview which seek out the manifestations of pathology in psychosocial space. The question then arises as to what is the relationship of these two technologies? Are they complementary or are they rivals?

This book can itself be seen as a manifestation of the desire to resolve this question. The human scientists cannot comment on the technical excellence of the new technologies for making the anatomical body legible, but they can – and do – challenge the unintended consequences of these technologies on the psychosocial space of the patient. The latter part of this chapter therefore offers some thoughts on the relationship between these two technologies.

TECHNOLOGIES OF VISIBILITY

First, a word of caution: the advent of the clinical technologies during the late eighteenth and early nineteenth centuries was marked by a lengthy period of consolidation, so similarly it might be expected that the new technologies for analysing psychosocial space will take several decades to assert themselves. It is therefore difficult to offer a proper judgement on their relationship with the older technologies in these relatively early years; nevertheless, it is possible to speculate that the new technologies seem to be 'winning' and that the old technologies are being tamed. Whether this means that the latter will eventually disappear as did the techniques of humoral medicine before them – only time will tell.

So, what sort of evidence can be advanced for the increasing dominance of the new technologies which might be characterised, following Foucault, as those of the 'confession'? The changing analysis of death over the last few decades provides a good illustration (Armstrong 1987).

One of the cardinal techniques of pathological medicine has been the post-mortem. The post-mortem has allowed the secrets of the body to be finally revealed to the medical eye. The findings could then be assigned to the patient's medical record as the truth about their death. These judgements, in their turn, were collated by the State and controlled through a system of death registration from the mid nineteenth century onwards. Thus, in Britain, from 1838, there is the beginning of a record of the causes of death of all individuals. Of course, in the early years these statements were rather vague and often unrelated to the notion of the pathological lesion, but during the twentieth century they have become increasingly focused on the precise cause of death. In sum, there is a long history of the application of increasingly sophisticated clinical and laboratory tests to the corpse to discover the true nature of its death.

However, during the last few decades a parallel analysis of death has emerged. Its origin can be dated quite precisely to the early 1960s. For millennia the chief mourners of a death had always have been the close friends and relatives of the deceased: in the early 1960s a fundamental inversion of this principle occurred when the chief mourners became the dying persons themselves. Perhaps the most well-known illustration of this shift is Kubler-Ross's description of the different stages which have come to mark the *rites de passage* of the dying patient (1969). It is now becoming increasingly common for the psychosocial space of the dying patient to be subjected to intense interrogation as patients are led to reveal their psychosocial lives to their medical or nursing attendant. Thus, there are now two parallel methods of exploring death. One relies on the necropsy and clinical techniques to establish the cause of death, the other uses a psychosocial technology to explore, through their dying, the truth of the patient. Are these simply complementary? They may be; but there is evidence that during the 1950s and 1960s, as the rival technologies emerged, a debate arose about the 'truth' of the statement of the cause of death recorded on the death certificate. A number of reports began to challenge the validity of causes of death recorded on death certificates, particularly following studies of the procedures through which clinicians and pathologists assigned a cause of death (Medical Services Study Group 1978). Thus necropsy findings, for nearly two centuries held to be the ultimate medical truth, are now seriously suspect. Does this mark a faltering in confidence in the old anatomical technologies which analyse the body, just as the newer approaches to the interrogation of death become more pervasive?

Another example comes from the field of diabetes where a number of technological advances in recent years has enabled the patients glycaemic state to be established with increasing certainty (Armstrong 1991). The glucometer allows instant and accurate readings of blood sugar to be taken by doctors, nurses and patients; and over the last decade the measurement of glycosylated haemoglobin has given diabetologists the means of establishing the patient's glycaemic state over the preceding several weeks. In the great tradition of making the body visible, both of these techniques have enabled diabetologists to gaze into the internal functioning of the body with increasing clarity.

Curiously, however, these techniques seem to have been compromised by patients' behaviour. A series of studies during the 1980s asked patients to keep a regular record of their blood glucose as recorded by a glucometer. Unknown to the patient, the glucometer also contained a memory chip which recorded the actual blood glucose as these patients measured and recorded their glycaemic state. The accounts from patients and glucometers were later shown to be widely discrepant (Mazze *et al.* 1984). Equally, the individual logs of glycaemic control maintained by patients were shown to be at considerable variance with their assumed glycaemic control from the measurement of glycosylated haemoglobin (Mazze *et al.* 1984). Diabetologists have been perplexed by these findings. They have been inclined to believe the findings from their technology, but this would appear to show that their patients are 'cheating' or 'lying' (Silverman 1987). In effect, this technology is in conflict with a different version of truth which is being manufactured in some way, and with a strange rationality, by the patient. One truth arises from a gaze to the interior of the body, but the other represents the view of the patient about what is happening in their own bodies. It is less a question of which is 'correct', more which will win; and it is quite clear that diabetologists are going to have to begin to explore the 'truth' of the patient's world view in more detail if they are to have any success in managing the illness.

CONCLUSION

The fact that a meeting on high technology medicine should involve so many 'human scientists', who according to their disciplinary affiliations have little direct knowledge of the workings of high technology medicine, adds support to the arguments presented above. Why is it that the technicians who build and operate the machines which form the basis of high technology medicine are requested to justify themselves to these human scientists? There are no parallel meetings at which social scientists have to justify their humanist concerns and actions in promoting a 'patient-centred' medicine. The reason seems clear. Despite the fact that the overt purpose of the meeting is to subject high technology medicine to a novel psychosocial analysis, everywhere one looks this is already occurring. Practitioners of high technology medicine cannot stir without being hit by the bricks of ethical analysis or psychological consequences or social context or economic opportunity cost. True, there is a nightmare scenario of untrammelled high technology medicine, but this simply serves to justify the demands of human scientists for this sort of medicine to be made subservient to a psychosocial perspective. The bad dream is working well: despite the rhetoric, high technology medicine is being well tamed.

REFERENCES

Armstrong, D. (1983), *Political Anatomy of the Body: Medical Knowledge in Britain in the Twentieth century*, Cambridge University Press

—— (1984), 'The patient's view', *Social Science and Medicine*, xviii, pp. 737–44

—— (1987), 'Silence and truth in death and dying', *Social Science and Medicine*, xxii pp. 651–7

—— (1991), 'The social context of technology in diabetes care: "compliance" and "control" ', In C. Bradley, P. D. Home, and M. J. Christie, (eds.), *The Technology of Diabetes Care*, Harwood, London

Cabot, R. C. (1938), *Physical Diagnosis* (12th edition), Bailliere Tindall, London

Foucault, M. (1973), *The Birth of the Clinic: An Archaeology of Medical Perception*, Tavistock, London

—— (1977), *Discipline and Punish: The Birth of the Prison*, Allen Lane, London

Kubler-Ross, E. (1969), *On Death and Dying*, Macmillan, New York

Lukes, S. (1973), *Individualism*, Blackwell, Oxford

McLeod, J. (ed.) (1976), *Clinical Examination* (4th edition), Churchill Livingstone, London

Mazze, R. S. *et al.* (1984), 'Reliability of blood glucose monitoring by patients with diabetes mellitus', *American Journal of Medicine*, lxxvii, pp. 211–17

Medical Services Study Group (1978), 'Death certification and epidemiological research', *British Medical Journal*, ii, p. 1065

Silverman, D. (1987), *Communication and Medical Practice: Social Relations in the Clinic*, Sage, London

Stevens, W.M. (1910), *Medical Diagnosis*, Lewis, London

Williams, R. (1976), *Keywords*, Fontana, London

15

Rehabilitating sick people: high technology and the reconstruction of normal possibilities

IAN ROBINSON

INTRODUCTION

[After being injured in an explosion] Brenda was rushed to the hospital and taken at once to the operating room where a team of surgeons attempted to save her life. [Although] . . . her brain and vital organs were functioning satisfactorily . . . the right side of her body had been completely mutilated . . . their only hope was to use replacement parts . . . They replaced her smashed ribs with . . . Vitallium metal . . . For her amputated right arm and right leg, they attached artificial limbs powered by nuclear energy . . . They implanted a glass eye [and] inside the glass eye they hid a sub-minature television camera. They fixed in place an ear . . . [and] in the ear opening, the surgeons placed a very sensitive, super-small microphone . . .

It was in school that Brenda most enjoyed her synthetic limbs and organs. In gym, of course, she could throw and kick farther, catch better, do more difficult gymnastic tricks, and win at almost any sports she tried . . . And in all her classes she could read an entire page at a single glance'.

(Berger 1978 pp. 3–4)

This quotation is 'faction' written by Berger to explore some current and future possibilities of bionic development in the late 1970s. Such images of bionic men and women have, over the past few years, captured the public imagination. Their construction of 'part flesh and blood, and part metal, plastic and wire' (Berger 1978 p. 4), knitted seamlessly together with advanced micro-electronics builds a 'new' out of an 'old' person. In this kind of story accidents are opportunities and disasters lead to successes. Functional abilities are hugely, indeed superhumanly, increased. Senses are made more acute and the bionic person becomes larger than life. Bionic components are conceived as both replaceable and extendable to other areas of (human) body malfunction. However the problems of, and images about, bionic people do not centre so much on technical issues of physical competence, but more on issues of personhood. Such issues are at the core of concern about the bionic self, and focus on the nature and intentions of the newly created person. For, in bionic fabrication, the 'person' appears to be contingent on this process rather than be able to condition or control it.

The reconstruction of people, through a range of technologies, has always been part of the agenda in the field of rehabilitation. The present frontiers of high technology research in bioengineering and rehabilitation engineering provide as fertile a source of bionic possibilities as is set out in Berger's account. They are, moreover, drawn from an extensive experimental clinical base of research. Conductive body implants as hearing aids (Browning 1990); functional electrical stimulation (FES) based mobility systems for paraplegic people (Marsolais 1985), later developed into functional neuromuscular stimulation (FNS) systems (Marsolais *et al.* 1990) using neural nets; myoelectric upper limbs for both adults and children, with FNS based electrical elbows (Sauter 1991; Hermansson 1991); robotic navigational and manipulative aides (Regalbuto *et al.* 1992); all illustrate the range of replacement mechanisms or body parts which are currently being developed for applications within the broad field of rehabilitation. These examples do not include a further area of rehabilitation focused research which has advanced rapidly in the last five years concerned with technologies for managing communication and a range of sensory deficits. Cheaper, smaller and more powerful micro-processor technologies, building on research in cybernetics and neuroscience, have led to the development of increasingly sophisticated speech synthesis systems; visual recognition systems for those with severe visual problems; an additional range of exotically engineered systems for managing complex hearing loss; systems for enhancing the sensitivity of touch, particularly for those with limbs operated with neuromuscular power; and other more general systems for managing proximate and remote personal communications.

The reconstruction of damaged individuals into 'bionic persons' from these technologies does not seem far away. Indeed all of the technologies are currently being clinically evaluated, and some are already in everyday use. Thus high technology based rehabilitation engineering has now moved to centre stage of the field of rehabilitation. However, the current major momentum behind these developments raises important issues about the nature of the rehabilitation process, as well as about the nature of sickness and disability and their perception and management.

THE IDEA OF REHABILITATION

The idea of rehabilitation has always been problematic to define either in terms of objectives or practices, and is becoming especially so in relation to rapidly developing technological imperatives. The field arose largely through pragmatic and crisis driven responses to the management of casualties during the first and second world wars (Gritzer and Arluke 1985). Acute medical models of intervention appeared to have relatively little salience to the longer term problems that were increasingly manifest amongst this large group. The medical process of rehabilitation, which was intended at first to assist in the renovation of soldiers for a speedy return to battle, became concerned as much with the care and reintegration of such war casualities into civilian, and then later into post-war life. This process of reintegration was not one that could be accomplished by physical remedies alone – a broad 'social cure' as well as a physical cure was needed. This realisation, together with other factors such as the increasing breadth of the potential clientele for rehabilitation; the complexity of their needs; the low status given to medical rehabilitationists; the correspondingly low level of prestige attached to the associated paramedical professions; and the limited and variable availability of resources, led to expedient rehabilitation ideologies and eclecticism in the wide range of associated practices.

The role of technology in rehabilitation until the 1960s – and much later in some cases – was generally as a modest resource to the aims and practices of others professionally concerned with the process. Rehabilitation technicians in Britain and the corresponding 'reconstruction aides' in the United States, became part of small numbers of centres which serviced the day to day problems of war veterans as well as some others whose disabilities resulted from civilian accidents or conditions. The technological skills that were practised were those that placed a premium on pragmatic low technology solutions to everyday problems. This was essentially a craft role, based on a cottage industry type of technology, in which expertise was learned 'on the job'. There was virtually no professional career or professional standing associated with the work. Tasks might involve making or adapting wheelchairs; making additional devices for those chairs, or their individual users, and building a wide range of everyday equipment on a 'made to measure' individual basis. Technicians or aides had relatively little or no formal specialist training for these specific tasks. Their main qualities were perceived to be the imaginative use of a wide range of local technologies, and their capacity to work effectively on an individual basis with the day to day problems of people with complex medical conditions.

However, a number of significant changes in the last two decades have led both to the reorientation of the field of rehabilitation, and more particularly to the transformation of the role of technology within it. Rapidly shifting demographic structures and patterns of disease in industrialised countries, have produced potentially more clients with age-related chronic conditions whose concerns and situation are radically different from those of young war casualties. Potential consumers of rehabilitation services have not only changed in numbers and characteristics, but also in their expectations about the level and type of professional support they require, as well as about their own role in the rehabilitation process (Robinson 1988). The size of the potential market of consumers for rehabilitation products and services has generated increasing commercial interest, which in its turn has promoted applied research. Greater involvement in the field from the core of the medical enterprise, and a corresponding rise in the status of rehabilitation medicine, has accompanied these changes.

As part of the transformation of the idea of rehabilitation the deployment of scientific knowledge in the form of rehabilitative technologies has proved of singular significance. In reflecting on the growth of interventionist engineering measures in this area Jacobs and Hughes (1990 p. 391), for example, echo the comments of many bioengineers in applauding the move in rehabilitation technologies from a craft to a science base, and the move from individual improvisation in techniques to the systematic application of rigorous biomechanical analysis. However, these and other robust views (James 1990) on the central role of engineering solutions in the rehabilitation process have been challenged by those who are fundamentally concerned about the axioms on which this technologically based interventionist stance is built, as well as about the very considerable commercial and research impetus behind recent developments.

Rehabilitation has in essence always been directed to remedying the differences (deficiencies) between assumed normal performances or capacities, and those of the rehabilitee. How those 'normal' performances or capacities are constructed, measured, and then remedied, forms the basis of a number of recent critiques of high technology rehabilitation. For example, Oliver argues that the extension of the role of science based medicine into the arena of rehabilitation confuses, and conflates sickness with disability (1990). The kinds of differences perceived between 'sick' and 'healthy' people are thus mirrored by those between 'disabled' and 'normal' people. And, further, the two sets of distinctions are treated in the same way, by being based in, and constantly referred back to a biomedical paradigm. Oliver implicitly asks the question if science based medicine has failed to cure the sickness, why should it be expected to redress the resulting functional disabilities? Moreover is the struggle for health over sickness the same as the struggle for normality over disability? Finkelstein recounts the dilemmas that the 'struggle for normality' posed for him in a spinal injury unit

> The result, for me, was endless soul destroying hours at Stoke Mandeville Hospital trying to approximate to able-bodied standards by 'walking' with calipers and crutches . . . Rehabilitation philosophy emphasises physical normality and, with this, the attainment of skills that allow the individual to approximate as closely as possible to able-bodied behaviour.
>
> (quoted in Oliver 1990 p. 54)

In this account Finkelstein points to one of the key factors which differentiates the management of disabilities in rehabilitation from the management of sickness in most areas of science based medicine – the unequivocally active role of all the participants in the process. This situation is formally recognised by those medically involved in rehabilitation. For example, Nichols notes that success 'depends [as much] on a patient's motivation, endurance and concentration as on physical capability.' (1980 p. 3). However for Nichols, as for other doctors (e.g. Licht 1968), the placing of such active involvement firmly within the doctor-patient relationship focused primarily on the detection and management of sickness, presents their patients with a paradox. On the one hand objectives to regain lost or deficient physical functions are established medically largely from outside the patient's frame of reference. On the other hand the patient is expected to become extraordinarily motivated and committed to those goals, and to pursue them actively at all times well outside the proper purview and (technically) the control of the doctor.

The difficulties inherent in this situation have led to such ideas as 'co-management' in rehabilitation where, acting outside conventional medical strategies, both client and professional staff could 'own' mutually agreed objectives and the means through which they may be accomplished (Wright 1983 Chapter 17). Albrecht also considers the negotiative aspects in rehabilitation important, although he recognises the problematic discrepancies of power and status between doctors (and other staff involved in the rehabilitation process) and the client in developing such a shared approach. He argues that (medical) control over the process is not as significant as it may appear, and that considerable agency is still vested in the client (1976 pp. 26–8).

Nonetheless the ways in which the goals of rehabilitation are constructed and practised fuses narrowly medical with broader social goals, both of which are based on prescriptive cultural understandings of normal and appropriate functioning. De Swaan sets this in context

> Society . . . enables its members to pursue their business as usual, and at the same time it compels them to do so. Whatever becomes a possibility for many turns into a necessity for everyone. If some physical defect or affliction can be cured, it must be. If the majority can read, the others thereby become illiterates who must also be taught to read and write . . . The conditions for achieving normality having been realised for everyone, its canons having become widely accepted, deviance is attributed solely to personal failure, to an individual handicap that should be corrected by a proper specialist.
>
> (1990 p. 1)

The reflection of these powerful beliefs and practices in the process of rehabilitation is demonstrated in the parallel and complementary development of the field along two broad tracks – specific medical interventions based on the technical recovery of physical functions, and retraining based on an educational approach to rehabilitation. This educational perspective both underpins medical interventions and links the rehabilitation process into more general social goals. The patient becomes the pupil, and the rehabilitation clinic becomes the schoolroom. Disability as a functional deficit deserving technical redress, becomes disability as a learning deficit requiring educational therapy. Learning to be 'normal' as Finkelstein has demonstrated in relation to spinal injury, and as de Swaan has indicated in relation to more general functional abnormalities, places onerous responsibilities on individuals subject to the rehabilitative process. In this respect the obligations socially imposed on sick patients to cooperate with medical advice to re-acquire health (Gerhardt 1989), seem modest compared to those socially imposed on people with functional disabilities to become 'normal'. The advent of high technology applications to functional problems appears to have increased rather than decreased these obligations.

RECONSTRUCTING NORMAL POSSIBILITIES

The rapidity with which high technology research in rehabilitation has grown in very recent years is indicated in the annual *Review of Rehabilitation Research and Development* produced by the Veterans' Administration in the United States. Between 1985 and 1990 the number of projects listed almost doubled to over 500. The *Review,* which incorporates research projects with a primary psychosocial focus as well as those targeted on equipment and other applications, showed an almost negligable increase in projects in the former category whilst those in the latter category increased markedly. Two major areas of high technology research – those focused on means of remedying neuromuscular disabilities, and on equipment concerned with managing personal communication and sensory deficits – showed the greatest growth.

Of particular interest is the impetus of research and clinical testing concerned with enhancing physical mobility by means of high technology strategies – especially through neuromuscular techniques – in those with spinal cord injuries. Oliver notes how the evaluation of success of rehabilitation programmes in this condition, where functional loss is so immediately and dramatically obvious, often hinge on the degree to which personal mobility – walking – is improved (1990 pp. 56–7). Indeed enabling 'paralysed' people to walk appears to have become the gold standard of high technology applications in this area.

Marsolais published a report in 1985 titled 'Walking restored in paralyzed man using electronic orthotics'. The associated work and its early and explicit promise to restore mobility has received wide publicity, and has encouraged continuing pilgrimages to Marsolais' laboratory by those seeking a restoration of their lost functions. However, a more detailed review of the extent of the 'restoration of walking' in the 1985 paper suggests a more equivocal situation. The FES mobility system, which was operating in a number of patients, had between 50 and 70 implanted electrodes working in an individual at any one time. The electrodes initially had a substantial failure rate although it decreased after the fourth month to 2–3 per cent each month. The patient who walked with the FES system appeared to possess some mobility already, which was then enhanced in various respects (for example, in stride length and speed) by the system. The context in which this occurred, and some of the system's more fundamental problems, were revealed by Solomonow *et al.* (1985). They note that their 'evaluation of several FES based walking prototypes . . . has revealed the weakness of the total FES approach to this problem'. In particular there were concerns about additional injuries from electrical or other malfunctions, and amongst 'the human factors' considered to be problematic in using FES systems was the requirement to suspend the patient from the ceiling for safety because the system resulted in the 'need for the patient to constantly lean forward, which is risky and uncomfortable' (p. 36). In summary Solomonow *et al.* argue that 'current [FES] prototype systems are still substantially remote from being practical and reliable for routine clinical application'(p. 36).

In a report on the same work five years later Marsolais and his colleagues had modified their title to read '*Functional tasks* restored in paralyzed man using electic orthotics' (1990, italics added). The report itself appears to make rather more modest claims for the current clinical effectiveness of the systems now being used, emphasising their capacity to enable all those with spinal cord injuries to stand, but to assist the walking of some others. However, optimism is expressed about the promise of the new (FNS) systems being based on artificial neural network technology (Abbas *et al.* 1990). In this work neural network pattern generators are being used to develop control mechanisms for activated neuromuscular systems. Jacobs and Hughes reflect the excitement felt in other areas of bioengineering in relation to these developments of 'hybrid orthoses [combining] biomechanically designed devices with functional electrical stimulation in the treatment of people with particular lesions of the spinal cord' (1990 p. 391).

The technological momentum associated with the development of orthoses for such purposes is also present in research on robotics in rehabilitation. Where functional deficiences are not easily remedied with orthoses applied to body surfaces or implanted in body structures, an alternative technical solution has been considered to be robot devices controlled in innovative ways, even by those with the most severe functional difficulties. For example Regulbato *et al.* (1992) optimistically describe the uses of the 'Hero 2000' robot for 'pick up and place' tasks, and for other manipulative assistance as part of the armoury of rehabilitative techniques. Selected surveys seemed to support this optimism by indicating positive attitudes towards robots and robotic devices. Prior found that 84 per cent of wheelchair users in his survey would consider buying a robotic arm for their wheelchair (1990). Englehardt *et al.* (1985) found a very high proportion of the staff and patients they studied in a Veterans' Administration Home Care Unit agreed with statements supporting the use of high technology equipment in this area. Thus 95 per cent agreed that 'computers have made living easier'; 86 per cent agreed that 'a robot would be useful in my job'; and 96 per cent agreed that 'robots have many useful applications'. They note that all respondents described robots as 'positive, valuable and useful', and the patients themselves were 'very positive' (p. 137).

Nonetheless some of the difficulties in incorporating such devices in everyday life, after testing in an institutional environment are noted by Hillman *et al.* (1991) in their survey of users of robots, who were unsure about the potential value of the systems. As they note, 'because the robot is a flexible device, the context in which it is introduced will affect the way it is perceived by potential users . . . the hospital environment does not fully reflect the situation in which the robots will be used' (p. 239). Another study of robot use in assisting therapy after stroke by Djikers *et al.* (1991) showed that both professional and staff and patients tended to focus on what the robot could *not* do, and were generally concerned with its deficiencies rather its capabilities. There was also some evidence in this study that robots were accepted (rather than welcomed) for only a short time, as their novelty value decreased and the their deficiences were more noticeable. Djikers *et al.* sum up their general view on current robots thus

> Any equipment that is complicated, difficult to set up, quick to break down, or provide feedback that is not understood, is not likely to be in use for long, even though it may have been accepted initially because of the glamour of high technology.
>
> (1991 p. 41)

Pullin and Gammie (1991) add further substantial caveats to what they see as the current enthusiasm for robots. They caution against excessive optimism, lest unrealistic and therefore disappointed expectations hamper development of the systems. They also note that it will only be simpler, less complex and less expensive systems that stand any chance of adoption in the rehabilitation process.

Thus reconstructing normal possibilities through the clinical application of high technology ideas in the areas of neuromuscular orthoses and robotics has been problematic. Although initial technical enthusiasm has been considerable, the complexities of the everyday situations in which the ideas would be applied, together with what are enigmatically described as 'human factors', have produced a far more circumspect view of the viability of the ideas.

USING HIGH TECHNOLOGY SOLUTIONS IN REHABILITATION

The understandable focus of high technology initiatives on the technical, to the neglect of the 'human' aspects of functional problems, embeds the resulting solutions in professional objectives. Even if technically competent solutions are developed for rehabilitative problems, their widespread use is conditioned by the extent to which solutions remain in this professional domain. Mann (1986) develops this theme in comparing the spread of two rehabilitation technologies – braille translation programmes and cybernetic artificial limbs. The former technology has now been widely disseminated and used, the latter technology has a very modest number of users compared to the potential clientele. He concludes that the spread of braille translation programmes has occurred precisely because of the separation of blind or visually impaired people from the medical system. Furthermore, the translation systems have been based on conventional non-specialist computer developments, and have thus benefited almost immediately from general technological improvements such as more efficient and powerful software and hardware, and their lower cost. On the other hand the development and fitting of advanced artificial limbs has remained part of the medical system involving surgery, rehabilitation, professional fitting, and associated therapy. At each stage of this process professional decision makers are involved and 'the milieu which the amputee finds him or herself in is more complex even than the health care system [at large]' (p. 4). Minnes and Stack (1990) in their review of the use by congenital amputees of the kinds of prostheses discussed by Mann appear surprised to find that 'contrary to expectation, provision of a prosthesis does not ensure its use' (p. 155), although they then expound a substantial range of 'human factors', as well as those associated with professional fitting and support, which plausibly account for this situation.

The extent to which rehabilitation technologies are separated from or are part of medical system has been taken up by other analysts. Batavia and Hammer's (1990) innovative study of users of such technologies points out that the most important factors for disabled people in deciding whether to use technologies are exactly those which guide other non-disabled users. Indeed a member of Batavia and Hammer's users' advisory panel commented that 'the most efficient test of whether to purchase a device is whether it has survived and flourished on the open market' (1990 p. 433). In the light of their review of other work, and the findings of their own study Batavia and Hammer themselves comment that

> The literature on rehabilitation engineering is replete with technical descriptions and analyses of the broad array of assistive devices that were intended to enhance the lives of people with disabilities... it contains no *comprehensive* analyses of the ultimate criteria by which such devices must be judged – the needs of the disabled consumer.
>
> (p. 425)

However it might be argued, even from Batavia and Hammer's own study, that it is precisely the focus on the 'disabled consumer' set apart from others and placed clearly within the medical system that has resulted in the variable, and generally low take-up of new rehabilitative technologies. A greater emphasis on the everyday utility of all kinds of technologies, for disabled and non-disabled people alike, may provide a more satisfactory base from which to develop particular variants for disabled users. Within this kind of paradigm *all* people are perceived to have functional problems in relation to socially sanctioned expectations which require the use of different technologies (for example employing toothbrushes to clean teeth; knives and forks to eat, and so on). We can therefore consider the rehabilitation process to focus on those who have a different *degree* of functional difficulty to others, but which is not different in *kind*. The 'Tools for Living' programme (BIB 1992) is one initiative seeking to extend and develop everyday (low) technologies for disabled people, with the similar and explicit aim of large markets and commercial viability to organisations developing technologies for less disabled people. Such an approach may also be viable for some micro-processor based technologies, as the example of the braille translation programme suggests.

CONCLUSION: HIGH TECHNOLOGY AND THE NATURE OF THE REHABILITATIVE PROCESS

The recent history of rehabilitation technologies has been replete with examples of sophisticated technical approaches to functional problems. However, the basic ambiguities which are associated with the idea of rehabilitation remain as they were. There is relatively little evidence that focusing on the technical redress of functional problems as the key to successful rehabilitation is the most profitable strategy. There appears to be little direct linkage between the amelioration of functional problems and positive personal or social outcomes (such as enhanced psychological status, greater social integration or more likelihood of employment). Indeed, one of the major current issues in this field is how, and in what ways, successful outcomes can be measured at all. This problem is compounded by difficulties in selecting potentially successful rehabilitees who, within the present rehabilitative process, are assumed to require an array of supportive motivational and attitudinal characteristics as well as remediable functional problems – the combination of which cannot easily be identified in individuals.

The issues posed by the difficulty of incorporating high technology solutions in the rehabilitative process warrant a reconsideration of the broader questions raised by Oliver (1990) and others. Extrapolating from his position, it could be argued that the current relative failure of high technology intiatives in this area has been for at least four reasons. First, that the majority of such interventions have been based on a narrow view of 'normality', which even in functional terms fails to take into account the diversity evident in the continuum which is 'normal' life. Second, such a focus has become embedded in and fused with the medicalisation of disability, improperly conflating it with sickness (and thus normality with health). Third, the 'technologising' of the solutions to disability has fundamentally located and confirmed that the problems are individual rather than arise from the context in which individuals operate. Therefore the focus has been on the deficiencies and motivations of the individual rather than on modifications to that individual's social or physical environment. And fourth, this approach has generally dis-empowered rather than empowered the individual through reinforcing the assymetry between professional and client, thereby making the possibility of active co-partnership in deciding rehabilitation objectives less likely.

However, it could be said that it is too easy to be overly pessimistic about the applicability of high technology research in the area of rehabilitation. For example, Locker and Kaufert (1988) remind us that whilst the use of most medical technologies is an optional process, for certain people sophisticated technologies are crucial to their survival. For some post-polio survivors ventilators are, as Locker and Kaufert put it, 'the breath of life'. For these people, and others such as those with heart pacemakers and implantable insulin delivery systems, reliance on these technologies has become a part of their existence. Nonetheless, even (perhaps especially) in these circumstances the use of such technologies occasions considerable concern, not least over their short and long term reliability, and the degree to which 'human factors' make a meaningful everyday life with them possible (Locker and Kaufert 1988; Pickup 1989). Thus these, and other more advanced technologies enumerated by Berger at the outset of this chapter – a number of which are being clinically evaluated – prompt profound doubts about their capacity to reconstruct even 'normal' possibilities in the near future, let alone create the exceptional capacities of bionic people.

REFERENCES

Abbas, J. A., Okunade, L. and Chizeck, H. J. (1990) 'Functional tasks restored in paralyzed man using electric orthotics: neural network controllers for FNS locomotion', on Department of Veterans' Affairs (1990), *Rehabilitation R & D Reports*, Supplement of *Journal of Rehabilitation Research and Development* , xxviii, pp. 121–2

Albrect, G. (1976), 'Socialisation and the disability process', in G. Albrecht (ed.), *The Sociology of Physical Disability and Rehabilitation*, University of Pittsburgh Press, pp. 3–38

Batavia, A. I. and Hammer, G. S. (1990), 'Towards the development of consumer based criteria for the evaluation of assistive devices', *Journal of Rehabilitation Research and Development*, xxvii, pp. 425–36

Berger, M. (1978), *Bionics*, Franklin Watts, New York

BIB (Brunel Institute for Bioengineering) (1992), *Tools for Living*, BIB, Brunel, The University of West London

Browning G. G. (1990), 'The British experience of an implantable, subcutaneous bone conduction hearing aid (Xiomed Audiant)', *Journal of Laryngology and Otology*, civ, pp. 534–8

Department of Veterans' Affairs (1990), *Rehabilitation R & D Reports*, Supplement of *Journal of Rehabilitation Research and Development* , xxviii

de Swaan, A. (1990), *The Management of Normality*, Routledge, London

Djikers, M. P., deBear, P. C., Erlandson, R. F., Kristy, K, Geer and D. M., Nichols, A. (1991), 'Patient and staff acceptance of robotic technology in occupational therapy', *Journal of Rehabilitation Research and Development*, xxviii, pp.33–44

Englehardt, K. G., Awad-Edwards, R., Haber, P., Wilson, D. and Van der Loos, M. (1985), Long-term health care applications for robotic technology', in Veterans' Administration, *Rehabilitation R & D Reports*, Department of Medicine and Surgery, Rehabilitation Research and Development Service, New York, pp. 136–37

Gerhardt U. (1989), *Ideas about Illness*

Gritzer, G. and Arluke, A. (1985), *The Making of Rehabilitation*, University of California Press, Berkeley

Hermansson, L. M. (1991), 'Structured training of children fitted with myoelectric prostheses,' *Prosthetics and Orthotics International*, xv, pp. 88–92

Hillman, M. R., Pullin, G. M., Gammie, A. R. et al. (1991), 'Clinical experience of rehabilitation robots', *Journal of Biomedical Engineering*, xiii, pp. 239–43

Jacobs, N. A. and Hughes, J. (1990), 'Advances in technology in prosthetics and orthotics', *Proceedings of the 5th Regional Conference of Rehabilitation International*, National Rehabilitation Board, Dublin, pp. 390–2

James, W. V. (1990), 'The provision of technical aids for the disabled', in *Proceedings of the 5th European Regional Conference of Rehabilitation International*, National Rehabilitation Board, Dublin, pp. 384–6

Licht, S. (1968), *Rehabilitation Medicine*, Waverly Press, Baltimore

Locker, D. and Kaufert, J. (1988), 'The breath of life: medical technology and the careers of people with post-respiratory poliomyelitis', *Sociology of Health and Illness*, x, pp. 23–40

Mann, R. W. (1986), 'Selected perspectives on a quarter century of rehabilitation engineering', *Journal of Rehabilitation Research and Development*, xxiii, pp. 1–6

Marsolais, E. B. (1985), 'Walking restored in paralyzed man using electronic orthotics', in Veterans' Administration, *Rehabilitation R & D Reports*, Department of Medicine and Surgery, Rehabilitation Research and Development Service, New York, pp. 178–9

Marsolais, E. B., Kobetic, R., Chizeck, H. J., Scheiner, A. and Jacobs, J. (1990), 'Functional tasks restored in paralyzed man using electric orthotics: FNS walking in paraplegics,' in Department of Veterans' Affairs (1990), *Rehabilitation R & D Reports*, Supplement of *Journal of Rehabilitation Research and Development*, xxviii, pp. 122–3

Minnes, P. M. and Stack, D. M. (1990), 'Research and practice with congenital amputees: making the whole more than the sum of the parts', *International Journal of Rehabilitation Research*, xiii, pp. 151–60

Nichols, P. J. R. (ed.) (1980), *Rehabilitation Medicine*, Butterworth's, London

Oliver, M. (1990), *The Politics of Disablement*, Macmillan, London

Pickup, J. C. (1989), 'Implantable insulin delivery systems', in D. F. Williams, (ed.), *Current Perspectives on Implantable Devices*, JAI Press, London, pp. 181–202

Prior, S. D. (1990), 'An electric wheelchair mounted robotic arm: a survey of potential users', *Journal of Medical Engineering Technology*, xiv, pp. 143–54

Pullin, G. and Gammie, A. (1991), 'Current capabilities of rehabilitation robots'. *Journal of Biomedical Engineering*, xiii, pp. 215–16

Regalbuto, M. A., Kroustrop, T. A. and Cheatham, J. B. (1992), 'Towards a practical mobile robotic aid system for people with severe disabilities', *Journal of Rehabilitation Research and Development*, xxix, pp. 19–26

Robinson, I. (1988), 'The rehabilitation of patients with long-term physical impairments', *Clinical Rehabilitation*, ii, pp. 339–47

Sauter, W. F. (1991), 'The use of electric elbows in the rehabilitation of children with upper limb deficiencies', *Prosthetics and Orthotics International*, xv, pp. 93–5

Solomonow, M., Shoji, H., D'Ambrosia, R. and Douglas, R. (1985), 'Electromechanical walking system for paraplegics', in Veterans' Administration, *Rehabilitation R & D Reports*, Department of Medicine and Surgery, Rehabilitation Research and Development Service, New York, pp. 36–7

Wright, B. A. (1983), *Physical Disability: A Psychosocial Approach*, Harper and Row, New York

16

Technology, medicine and the psychosocial context: the case of psychoneuroimmunology

MARGOT L. LYON

INTRODUCTION: TECHNOLOGY AND MEDICINE

Technology constitutes the instruments and practices of particular types of knowledge. Technologies are therefore but forms or practical manifestations of knowledge. Medical technologies, by definition, operate in terms of views of the subject (i.e., the person or patient) commensurate with the particular domains of medical knowledge from which that technology arose, or which seek to apply that technology. Thus, the research foundation of a particular technology and the epistemology of medical science are articulated at the level of medical diagnosis and treatment. This means that the view of the person inherent in technology is conceived through the perspectives derived from molecular, cellular, organ, or system levels or even population levels, if we include large data bases as a form of technology. These different perspectives on the subject are embedded in particular technologies, as for example in screening techniques derived from molecular genetics, or the development of artificial body parts. Questions of what measures are used in determining the value and the efficacy of medical technologies, however, must be answered with reference to the larger social, political and economic framework within which medicine is practised. Technology itself does not measure anything external to it, that is, outside the knowledge which gave it form; whatever perspectives it has on the 'social' are likely to be implicit, embedded in the technological form itself. But the consequences or implications of a medical technology extend into social and economic and therefore even political considerations. To pose the question of this larger social context and therefore the extra-medical implications of any particular technology necessarily requires a step outside that framework.

All of this leads to the importance of context, and therefore to questions about what might be called the 'situated organism'. The concept of 'situatedness' is crucial here, for it indicates the range of possibilities in the 'connections' between an organism and its environment. We are reminded of the impact of its situation on the organism, the complex nature of this interrelationship, and how it is to be conceptualized and treated. Thus, questions that are grounded in perspectives which go beyond the merely technical have serious implications for the types of knowledge generated in and for medical practice. My concern in this chapter is to ask such questions using the example of a 'new' and growing domain of knowledge in medical research, that is, the field of psychoneuroimmunology (PNI). PNI attempts to examine the interrelationships between social and psychological situatedness and immune function.

High technology, by definition, is seen to intervene primarily on a physical level, on material substance. Yet, findings in PNI and related fields show that this 'substance' may be seen to operate at levels not readily integrated, conceptually or theoretically, into the 'physical domain', that is, those aspects of embodiment which remain conceptually isolated as part of social or psychological domains. Yet, medical 'intervention' is indeed conceived, by those influenced by the findings of PNI or similar research, to operate on all levels including these so-called 'non-material' ones.

Medical knowledge arises out of the same socio-cultural–scientific research context as the particular objects and practices we call 'high technology medicine', and carries with it implications for how we think about health, illness, and healing. But new scientific measures which make possible correlations across both the 'physical' and 'non-physical' social or psychological domains, also entail a wider perspective for the understanding of the ontology of health and illness, and therefore the foundations of medical knowledge and the technologies which arise from it. The field of PNI provides an ideal arena in which to consider such questions. PNI can therefore be seen to generate new questions about the relationship of particular forms of knowledge to particular technologies and vice versa. In the following, the example of the study of emotion is used both to condense and to help clarify the issues raised by the development of PNI and their implications for the nature and practice of medicine.

WHAT IS PSYCHONEUROIMMUNOLOGY?

PNI is an emerging, interdisciplinary field concerned with the interrelationships between the central nervous system, the endocrine system and the immune system: systems which have heretofore been treated independently both conceptually and methodologically. PNI purports to go beyond conventional biomedical perspectives and to be concerned with fundamental questions about the relationship of thought, feeling, and action to immune system function and therefore to health and illness. Its conception raises again, in a new technical context, questions about the most basic concerns of medicine, that is, questions of the nature of healing and the nature of therapy (Lyon 1993).

The roots of PNI lie in many disciplines including the neurosciences, endocrinology, immunology, psychology, psychiatry, as well as epidemiology and ethology (Locke *et al.* 1985). Other terms may be used, such as psychoimmunology, behavioural immunology, neuro-endocrine-immunology (NEI), the ponderous psychoneuro-endocrino-immunology, and neuro-immunomodulation (NIM). The term PNI is perhaps most prevalent, particularly in the United States, with widespread use in both scientific and popular literature (Cousins 1989). Its construction gives emphasis to psychological or behavioural dimensions (DiLeo and Strait 1990, p. 307). Neuroimmunomodulation is the preferred term for a number of American and European scientists on the grounds that it is simpler and yet can encompass through its use of the term 'neuro' all manner of nervous system–immune system interactions including the psychological (Spector 1987; 1992).[1] Its significance is reflected in the title of one organization in the field, the International Society for Neuroimmunomodulation (ISNIM). Some scholars deny the validity of a single term to encompass such diverse disciplinary areas, and prefer to use a descriptive phrase such as 'brain, behaviour, and immunity', as in the title used for the first major journal in the field of PNI, founded in 1987 by Robert Ader. Others deny the need for a new term at all; rather, they insist that the boundaries of fields such as psychobiology, psychosomatics, or behavioural medicine, can encompass new developments. Ader, for example, sees PNI as a subdivision of psychosomatic or psychophysiological phenomena, founded on the common premise of mind–body interconnectedness (1987, p. 357). None of the terms make clear the place of the societal domain except apparently to subsume it within 'behavioural' or 'psychological' forms.

The impetus for the emergence of PNI is said to lie in research findings in a number of fields requiring an integrative approach to immune system functioning. Such an approach must consider

'immune processes as an integrated part of the organism's psychological adapation to its environment' (Ader 1981a, p. xxi). PNI is heralded
as a new paradigm of health and illness and has a high profile in the
media and is a frequent topic for public workshops and lecture series.
It also figures much in popular publishing in the health field, and
research findings are often re-read through the lens of various New
Age interests.

According to Herbert Spector, a neurophysiologist in the Division
of Fundamental Neurosciences of the National Institutes of Health in
the United States, it is one of the fastest growing areas of modern
medical research; in the United States in 1990, there were over 200
grants in the area funded through various sections of the National
Institutes of Health (Spector 1990, p. 382). It is thus an area of
potential career development in a competitive medical research funding market. One of the first conferences on NIM in the United States
was held at the University of Kentucky in May of 1983 (Melnechuk
1983). A few months later in October another conference on the
neural modulation of immunity was held in Belgium organized by
Roger Guillemin of the Salk Institute and others (Melnechuk 1984,
p. 56). The first international workshop on NIM was held in the
United States in 1984 (Spector 1985). The first compilation of works
in the area, edited by Robert Ader, was published in 1981 under
the title of *Psychoneuroimmunology*. The second, published in 1985,
comprised proceedings of the NIM conference in Belgium held in
October, 1983 (Guillamin *et al.* 1985). Also published in 1985 was
the book comprising a compilation of key articles entitled *Foundations
of Psychoneuroimmunology* edited by Locke *et al.*

The history of the field is seen to lie in work, mainly on conditioning, undertaken in earlier decades of this century at the Pasteur
Institute in Paris and in the Soviet Union. It was found that responses
of the immune system could be behaviourally conditioned through
classical Pavlovian conditioning techniques. This research raised profound questions about the interrelationships and interaction of
psychological and physiological domains.[2] Robert Ader, a psychiatrist,
and Nicholas Cohen, a microbiologist, continued and advanced
research through their work on the immune conditioning of rats
(1975).

Research on conditioning is only one approach to the study of
central nervous–immune system interaction. There are many other
directions and levels from which research on the inseparability of
psychobiological processes may proceed, as can be deduced from the
number of fields said to contribute to PNI and the types of research
generated within them.[3] There are vast differences in disciplinary
orientation between works such as an early paper on emotional con-

flict and immune response in rheumatoid arthritis by the psychologist, Moos, and the psychiatrist, Solomon (1964), and current papers on molecular biology and psychopharmacology (Spector 1990, p. 382). Immune function is now seen to be potentially located at all sites of the body through the action of certain cells and complex molecules. These are seen to act as 'messengers' between central nervous and immune systems and thus to modulate the activity of both (Institute of Medicine 1989). This activity has been referred to as a 'psychosomatic network' (Pert 1984; Camara and Danao 1989).

Psychoneuroimmunology, in defining itself as going beyond conventional biomedical perspectives, is concerned with the relationships between behaviour and physiology in a fundamental sense. An integrationist perspective is required, at least if PNI is to address the interrelationships between very different domains. Yet, while PNI fosters research about connections between quite different categories of phenomena, it tends to maintain the given categories of knowledge within the constituent disciplines. For example, while research on the mechanisms and roles of regulatory functions between central nervous and immune systems can proceed on any number of levels, problems arise when what is meant by the central nervous system is seen to encompass 'mind', a concept which is very differently understood from that of 'immune system': 'The immune system is understood in sufficient detail to measure the limiting factors in responsiveness with precision, while 'mind' is a collection of subjective and objective events and processes: i.e., emotions, stress, cognition (conscious and unconscious), conditioning, volition, etc.' (Guillemin *et al.* 1985, p. vi). The authors continue: '[t]his disparity would be sufficient reason to treat the problem circumspectly were not the effects of "mind" on immune reactivity so dramatic and paradoxical that the urge to understand becomes irresistible' (*ibid.*).

Psychoneuroimmunologic models or approaches which are alternative to the dualistic and reductionist model of conventional biomedicine[4] might be said to fall into two main areas. The first is what might be termed a psychosomatic or psychodynamic approach which works from psychological phenomena and explores how these may be linked to somatic changes. This approach is characteristic of much of the work undertaken in psychology and psychiatry and seems to be conceptualized in terms of the 'role' of behavioural factors in immune response. In effect, those using this perspective continue to explore correlations between the two domains through measures of immune function (for example, Glaser *et al.* 1987). The second approach focuses on the molecular level as the primary locus of psychoneural phenomena and works to build models of cellular communication which are said to obviate distinctions between mind and body.[5] Such an approach focuses instead on the possibility and mechanisms of functional parallels and communication between various levels of the organism, though one might say that the category of 'mind' is eliminated here, rather than the distinction between mind and body being obviated. This raises the problem that PNI tends to see 'mind' as the point of intersection of individual with the social world and therefore to give primacy to psychological forms as intermediary between body and environment.

The division between these two approaches, however, is primarily heuristic for each area would encompass a number of different perspectives, but it does make a point about different levels of analysis. The problem is, of course, to articulate a general framework within which each type of approach can be considered. Some attempts at linking cognitive and biological levels by treating each as information and assuming transformations between the two domains have been made through the application of systems and information theory to medicine (for example Temoshok 1983; Foss 1989). Further, models drawn from non-linear dynamics and the study of self-organizing systems are being brought to bear on the broader understanding of the body in context (for example, Stewart and Varela 1989; Vaz and Faria 1990; Yates 1987).

The nature of PNI, of course, cannot be discussed in the abstract, independent of its institutional embodiment. Although there are a number of interdisciplinary programmes in PNI in existence, researchers generally work from within their own disciplines. Such disciplinary specialization has implications for the nature of the models and measurements used in the design and application of research. Current intellectual determinants, for example, derive from biomedicine and its emphasis on molecular level research. Further, funding is also affected by institutional and disciplinary constraints, as well as larger political and economic factors. Broad collaborative research projects necessarily require special funding arrangements. All such constraints work to shape the development of the field.

The research and institutional contexts mentioned above have an impact on the potential clinical implications of developments in PNI. Questions need to be asked regarding the implications of these contexts for the reconceptualization of the structure of medicine and medical practice. Ader states that 'the functional significance of these links between the brain and the immune system remains to be determined' and acknowledges the problem of application of PNI within clinical settings. However, he does make some partial suggestions (1987, pp. 357–8). Ader *et al.* (1987, p. 1) state:

> Studies of isolated and interacting components within any given system

are necessary and critical for an understanding of that part of the adaptive apparatus. They are not sufficient, however, to describe the mechanisms by which adaptation may be achieved or compromised in an individual faced with the challenges that exist in the real world. Our current understanding of immunology is not sufficient to explain why allergic reactions can be precipitated by immunologically neutral but emotionally potent stimuli; why warts can be made to disappear under hypnosis; why the social environment can determine the individual's response to superimposed infectious diseases.

These comments seem to suggest the need to refocus attention away from the cellular and molecular manifestations of immune functioning as the primary locus of research and to give more attention to larger social and social interactional components. Ader *et al.* call for an increased understanding of immune functioning in context, noting that 'the strategies of the behavioural and neurosciences may have to be modified in consideration of the special nature of immune responses, and the strategies of immunology may have to be modified in consideration of the psychobiological setting within which immune responses occur' (1987, p. 2). What is needed are 'appropriately designed studies of psychosocially induced changes in the etiopathogenesis of the particular disease process under study' (Ader 1987, p. 358), but Ader acknowledges that the understanding of the mechanisms may not be sufficient to make such studies possible. Thus, except for an assumed increase in and refinement of awareness of the importance of a person's subjective state in immune functioning, which does little to clarify the already confused concept of mind in psychoneuroimmunological models, there has been relatively little systematic exploration in the scientific literature regarding the implications of PNI for the nature and structure of medical practice. There are an increasing number of carefully controlled studies which have incorporated attention to and measurement of the psychological state of individuals including the working toward the enhancement of 'positive' emotion states (for example, Fawzy *et al.* 1990, Parts I and II). There are also a wide range of more popular accounts written by both researchers in the field and laypersons (for example, Locke and Colligan 1986; Pelletier 1977; Achterberg 1985).

The general difficulties of a scientific engagement with such topics by PNI, despite the implications of its own research, is a reflection of larger intellectual issues in both the natural and social sciences. There remains a conceptual dualism in PNI in its attempts to incorporate both psychosocial and biological explanatory frameworks. This, in practice, leads towards reduction either to psychologically, or to physiologically grounded explanation, the very reduction that PNI as an interdisciplinary field appears to conceptually deny. The basis of this dualism lies in the problem of how to conceptualize both the subjective and the biological foundations of existence within one explanatory model.

CONCEPTUAL DUALISM IN THE BIOLOGICAL AND SOCIAL SCIENCES

The root of the divide between the natural and the social sciences, which we have seen reflected in developments in PNI, is generally attributed to so-called Cartesian dualism after Descartes' distinction between body, mind, soul. However, the seeking of present day conceptual categories in long past historical contexts is often spurious. The usefulness or persistence of certain categories may be a function of a quite different historical or intellectual context and the categories themselves may now serve quite different meanings. For example, Brown (1989), in an article tracing the origins of the notion of Cartesian dualism in psychosomatic medicine, points to the importance of the functional interaction of mind and body in Descartes' own writings and in the medicine of his time. He points out that it was during the nineteenth century, long after Descartes' time, that real changes in medical theory occurred (p. 328): 'Only at that late date were neoclassical conceptions abandoned and broadly replaced by views based on anatomical localism, cellular pathology, biochemical mechanism, and microbiological etiology – each fragmenting the notion of organismic totality implicit in humoral and posthumoral physiology.'

Medicine was further fragmented through specialization by bodily systems and organs, and developments in diagnostic medical techniques further removed doctors from patients. These developments effectively separated mind from body in medical theory. Reaction to these changes in the early decades of the twentieth century led eventually to the rise of psychosomatic medicine and related subspecialties (Brown 1989, p. 328). But psychosomatic medical specialists themselves, whose training is mainly in psychiatry and psychoanalysis, are caught up in dualism by virtue of their role in institutional medicine, that is, in order to work within biomedicine they must give both conceptual and practical ground to biomedicine (Brown 1989, p. 330).

Taking the context beyond medicine, the late nineteenth and early twentieth centuries saw the reproduction of particular dualisms or distinctions such as body/mind, nature/culture, biology/society which became crucial in 'establishing and legitimating an intellectual division of labour between the natural and the social sciences' (Benton 1991, p. 9). Developments in early twentieth century biology which provided the foundations of this specialization in medicine, for example, in genetics and molecular biology, were also responsible for encouraging further divisions between the biological and the human sciences. The subjective foundations of existence became the province of the social sciences and the somatic the province of the biological sciences.

There continue to be voices for the integration of body and mind, and of biological and social perspectives, from within both the natural and the social sciences (see Benton 1991; Lyon 1990, for example). Psychosomatic and behavioural medicine, psychobiology, psychology, and the current models coming from PNI represent attempts to pursue this integration. Within the social sciences and humanities, a concern with the question of the interrelationship of body and mind originates chiefly in philosophy, particularly the area of phenomenology, in certain areas in linguistics, in anthropology, especially critical medical anthropology (Lock and Gordon 1988), and in some areas of sociology, including sociological research on emotion.

There has been a recent re-emphasis on phenomenological approaches in anthropology and linguistics which emphasize embodiment as the basis of experience and hence of the formation of conceptual categories. Mark Johnson (1987), for example, explores how basic concepts such as containment, force, and balance arise from bodily experiences. These structures provide the basis for metaphorical elaborations which generate meaning in many cognitive domains (Johnson 1987, p. 65). The body is an active agent in the apprehension and construction of the world. For example, Johnson sees the 'bodily experience of balance as an activity' and states that it is 'an activity we learn with our bodies and not by grasping a set of rules or concepts. First and foremost, balancing is something we do. . . Balancing is a preconceptual bodily activity that cannot be described propositionally by rules' (1987, p. 74). Johnson extends the discussion of the experience of balance as in learning to ride a bicycle to the notion of systemic balance, also grounded in our bodies: 'There is too much acid in the stomach, the hands are too cold, the head is too hot, the bladder is distended, the sinuses are swollen, the mouth is dry. In these and numerous other ways we learn the meaning of lack of balance or equilibrium' (1987, p. 75).

Although it was not Johnson's aim to explore bodily correlates and their implications in detail, such a discussion of systemic balance can be extended to consider more fundamental structures of the body and how they function together. For example, Johnson, in order to suggest the importance of systemic balance in the larger sense, shows how the cultural notion of 'emotional balance' is both grounded in bodily experience and linked to more abstract notions of balance in reason, law, mathematics, etc. (1987, pp. 87–90, 95–6). One could draw parallels between the more conventional phenomenological understanding of the links between bodily experience and cognitive categories, and the understanding of the interrelationship between bodily being and the psychosocial world in a more profound physiological sense. For example, research on behaviourally conditioned immune response might be said to involve the notion of systemic balance operating simultaneously in both physiological (including neuroendocrine and immune functions) and cognitive domains. Freund (1990, p. 463) uses Johnson's work in making a similar and important point when he sees disease as an expression of a 'lack of coherence' which is somatically expressed.

EMOTION, MEDICINE, AND THE SITUATING OF THE BODY

Social and biological scientists are thus each subject to the problems associated with the conceptual gap between the so-called natural and social sciences. The study of emotion represents and condenses these problems as emotion is *both* biological and cognitive. Because emotion unavoidably impinges on both 'body' and 'mind', it provides a key theoretical area for the interdisciplinary development of models which can simultaneously encompass both biological and cognitive domains (Lyon and Barbalet 1994). The problem of category differences and the crudeness of 'measures' or 'models' in each domain, here immune function and emotion, is a difficult one, however. Johnson shows us the body is 'in' the mind, and argues for an embodied understanding of meaning. Likewise, we need an understanding of the 'body in the mind' which can also encompass the social and cultural contexts of embodiment, and the implications of these contexts in bodily being and agency, both external and internal. The phenomenon of emotion (along with its cognitive dimensions) can be said to encompass this 'being in the world' of the individual. It can therefore encompass the social and cultural contexts within which individuals develop, act, and are acted upon.

If the study of emotion is to provide a 'bridge' between cognitive and biological domains, it needs to work to demonstrate and clarify the interrelationships between physiology and emotion. In fact, there are a number of researchers whose work clearly links bodily, social, and psychological processes, including early sources such as Darwin (1872) writing on the expression of emotion, and Elias (1939) on the relationship of social structure and the experience of emotion. More recent studies include those of Ekman (1990); Ekman *et al.* (1983); Kemper (1978; 1987; 1990); Levenson *et al.* (1990); Papanicolaou (1989) and Scheff (1983; 1988), among others. Such writers go beyond the ways in which 'emotion' is typically used, which even in much of the literature in the sociology of health and illness is grounded in medical models. For example, the work on social stressors tends to be mechanistic and static, merely demonstrating correlations between emotion and changes in body function.[6] And, in the social and cultural constructionist approaches to emotion typical of much of social science, there is a tendency towards reduction of a comparable – but cultural – kind in the form of demonstrating how particular social or cultural contexts 'produce' or 'reproduce' the meaning of health and illness in a manner which is cut off from its bodily foundations.

One possibility for the bridging of bodily, social and psychological domains, is new perspectives arising in interdisciplinary research in areas such as PNI and theoretical immunology more generally, as well as perspectives arising in the study of embodiment and emotion within the social sciences. These may well generate a fundamental rethinking of the interrelationship of the social and neurophysiological, and thus eventually lead to accounts of the import of affective and social factors at least as complex as those of biology. The study of emotion provides one research route through which such perspectives can be developed. And, should the importance of 'situated representations of the organism' be acknowledged in medicine, a field such as PNI may provide an arena for research grounded in perspectives far beyond conventional biomedical ones.

Such speculation will remain theoretical and utopian if we fail to consider also its place in the context of the political economy of biomedicine and science, as well as social science. The politics of health, for instance, raises such questions as the source of the health of individuals and communities, the distinct and relative contributions of the provision of medical services, and the question of the nature of those services themselves. These must be considered in the context of practices relating to the larger environment including economic and social factors. The implications of research on complex interactions of physical and psychosocial phenomena would indicate a broader and potentially more political approach to health and illness. For the moment, complex, multi-factorial, epidemiological studies using large data bases may be more effective in answering questions about health and illness in social, psychological, and environmental context, as well as providing clues as to directions for future research, than more limited biomedical studies.

It was stated at the beginning of the chapter that one of the problems in fields such as PNI is how to articulate the operation of biological 'substance' at levels not yet conceptually or theoretically integrated into the 'physical domain,' that is, those aspects of embodiment which continue to be conceptually isolated as part of social or psychological domains. This, in turn, raises the question of intervention, for it, too, must be conceived to operate on all levels including so-called 'non-material' ones. Particular technologies may, nevertheless reveal non-reducible levels of organization. These, as Benton puts it, 'render[s] thinkable an extension of the idea of "levels" to include psychological and social processes and mechanisms whilst continuing to recognize these same processes and mechanisms as constituting discrete causal orders in their own right' (1991, p. 20). Neurophysiology, ethology and developmental biology are cited by Benton as offering 'insights into the mechanisms underlying the powers, liabilities and dispositions of persons considered as living organisms, as well as non-human animals' (1991, p. 20–1). Finally, it should be added that the study of emotion offers real possibilities in the integration of bodily and social domains.

NOTES

1 See also Solomon 1985 for a list of terms and their origins.

2 See Locke *et al.* 1985; Ader 1981a; Spector and Korneva 1981 for historical summaries.

3 See Locke and Hornig-Rohan 1983 for a survey of five different areas of research between 1976 and 1982.

4 See Engel 1977 and Brown 1989 for critiques and discussion of the role of so-called mind-body dualism in medicine; Lyon 1993 for discussion of dualism in PNI.

5 See Melnechuk 1989 for review of some approaches aired in 1988 at a conference of leading figures in PNI.

6 See Freund 1990, p. 454 for discussion.

REFERENCES

Achterberg, Jeanne (1985), *Imagery in Healing: Shamanism and Modern Medicine*, New Science Library, Boston

Ader, Robert (ed.) (1981a), *Psychoneuroimmunology*, Academic Press, New York (1981b), 'A historical account of conditioned immunobiologic responses', in Robert Ader (ed.), *Psychoneuroimmunology*, Academic Press, New York, pp. 321–54 (1987), 'Clinical implications of psychoneuroimmunology: commentary', *Journal of Developmental nd Behavioral Pediatrics*, VIII (6), pp. 357–8

Ader, Robert and Cohen, Nicholas (1975), 'Behaviorally conditioned immuno-suppression', *Psychosomatic Medicine*, XXXVII, pp. 333–40

Ader, Robert, Cohen, Nicholas, and Felten, David (1987), 'Brain, behavior, and immunity', *Brain, Behavior, and Immunity*, 1(1), pp. 1–6

Benton, Ted (1991), 'Biology and social science: why the return of the repressed should be given a (cautious) welcome', *Sociology*, XXV(1), pp. 1–29

Brown, Theodore M. (1989), 'Cartesian dualism and psychosomatics', *Psychosomatics*, XXX(3), pp. 322–31

Camara, Enrico G. and Danao, Theresa C. (1989), 'The brain and the immune system: a psychosomatic network', *Psychosomatics*, XXX(2), pp. 140–6

Cousins, Norman (1989), *Head First: The Biology of Hope*, E.P. Dutton, New York

Darwin, Charles (1872), *The Expression of the Emotions in Man and Animals*, Philosophical Library, New York

DiLeo, Joseph and Strait, Glenn Carroll (1990), 'Mapping the wisdom of the body', *The World and I*, June

Ekman, Paul (1990), 'The argument and evidence about universals in facial expressions of emotion', in H. Wagner and A. Manstead (eds.), *Handbook of Social Psychophysiology*, John Wiley & Sons Ltd, Chichester, pp. 143–64

Ekman, Paul, Friesen, Wallace V. and Levenson, Robert W. (1983), 'Autonomic nervous system activity distinguishes among emotions', *Science*, CCXXI, pp. 1208–10

Elias, Norbert (1978 (1939)), *The Civilizing Process: The History of Manners*, Basil Blackwell, Oxford

Engel, G.L. (1977), 'The need for a new medical model: a challenge for biomedicine', *Science*, CXCVI, pp. 129–36

Fawzy, F.I., Cousins, N., Fawzy, N., Kemeny, M., Elashoff, R. and Morton, D. (1990), 'A structured psychiatric intervention for cancer patients: Part I', *Archives of General Psychiatry*, XLVII, pp. 720–5

Fawzy, F.I., Kemeny, M., Fawzy, N., Elashoff, R., Morton, D., Cousins, N. and Fahey, J. (1990), 'A structured psychiatric intervention for cancer patients: Part II', *Archives of General Psychiatry*, XLVII, pp. 729–35

Foss, Laurence (1989), 'The challenge to biomedicine: a foundations perspective', *The Journal of Medicine and Philosophy*, XIV, pp. 165–91

Freund, Peter E.S. (1990), 'The expressive body: a common ground for the sociology of emotions and health and illness', *Sociology of Health and Illness*, XII(4), pp. 452–77

Glaser, R., Rice, J., Sheridan, J., Fertel, R., Stout, J., Speicher, C., Pinsky, D., Lotur, M., Post, A., Beck, M. and Kiecolt-Glaser, J. (1987), 'Stress-related immune suppression: health implications', *Brain, Behaviour, and Immunity*, I, pp. 7–20

Guillemin, Roger, Cohn, Melvin and Melnechuk, Theodore (1985), Preface, in Roger Guillemin, Melvin Cohn and Theodore Melnechuk (eds.), *Neural Modulation of Immunity* (Proceedings of an international symposium held in Brussels, October 27 and 28, 1983) Raven Press, New York, pp. v–vi

Institute of Medicine (Division of Health Sciences Policy and Division of Mental Health and Behavioral Medicine) (1989), *Research Briefing: Behavioral Influences on the Endocrine and Immune Systems*, National Academy Press, Washington, D.C.

Johnson, Mark (1987), *The Body in the Mind*, University of Chicago Press

Kemper, Theodore D. (1978), *A Social Interactional Theory of Emotions*, John Wiley & Sons, New York

(1987), 'How many emotions are there? Wedding the social and the autonomic components', *American Journal of Sociology*, XCIII(2), *pp. 263–89*

(1990), Social Structure and Testosterone: Explorations of the Socio-Bio-Social Chain, Rutgers University Press, New Brunswick

Levenson, Robert W., Ekman, Paul and Friesen, Wallace V., (1990), 'Voluntary facial action generates emotion-specific autonomic nervous system activity', *Psychophysiology*, XXVII(4), pp. 363–84

Lock, Margaret and Gordon, Deborah R. (eds.) (1988), *Biomedicine Examined*, Kluwer Academic Publishers, Dordrecht

Locke, Steven and Hornig-Rohan, Mady (1983) *Mind and Immunity: Behavioral Immunology: An Annotated Bibliography 1976–1982* Institute for the Advancement of Health, New York

Locke, Steven, Ader, R., Besedovsky, H., Hall, N., Solomon, G., Strom, T. and Spector, N.H. (1985), *Foundations of Psychoneuroimmunology*, Aldine, New York.

Locke, Steven and Colligan, Douglas (1986), *The Healer Within: The New Medicine of Mind and Body*, E.P. Dutton, New York

Lyon, Margot L. (1990), 'Order and healing: the concept of order and its importance in the conceptualization of healing', *Medical Anthropology*, XII(3), pp. 249–68

(1993), 'Psychoneuroimmunology: the problem of the situatedness of illness and the conceptualization of healing', *Culture, Medicine and Psychiatry*, XVII, pp. 77–97.

Lyon, M.L. and Barbalet, J.M. (1994), 'Society's body: emotion and the "somatization" of social theory', in T. Csordas (ed.), *The Body as Existential Ground of Culture*, Cambridge University Press

Melnechuk, Theodore (1983), 'Neuroimmunomodulation: conference report', *Advances*, I(1), pp. 29–31

(1984), 'Neural modulation of immunity: conference report, *Advances*, I(4), pp. 56–9

(1989), 'New models of health, illness, and disease: implications of psychoneuroimmunology', unpublished report of a conference, March 10–13, Lake Arrowhead, California

Papanicolaou, A.C. (1989), *Emotion: A Reconsideration of the Somatic Theory*, Gordon and Breach, New York

Pelletier, Kenneth (1977), *Mind as Healer, Mind as Slayer*, Dell Books, New York

Pert, Candace B., Ruff, M.R., Weber, A.J. and Herkenham, M. (1984), 'Neuropeptides and their receptors: a psychosomatic network', *Journal of Immunology*, CXXXV, pp. 820s–826s

Scheff, Thomas J. (1983), 'Toward integration in the social psychology of emotions', *Annual Review of Sociology*, IX, pp. 333–54

(1988), 'Shame and conformity: the deference-emotion system', *American Sociological Review*, LIII, pp. 395–406

Scherer, Klaus R. and Ekman, Paul (eds.) (1984), *Approaches to Emotion* , Lawrence Erlbaum Associates, Hillsdale, N.J.

Solomon, George F. (1985), 'The emerging field of psychoneuroimmunology', *Advances*, II(1), pp. 6–19

Solomon, George F. and Moos, Rudolf H. (1964), 'Emotions, immunity and disease: a speculative theoretical integration', *Archives of General Psychiatry*, XI, pp. 657–764

Spector, Herbert Novera (1985), 'Information explosions in an old–new research domain', in J.M. Cruse and R.E. Lewis, Jr (eds.), *The Year in Immunology*, S. Karger, Basel, pp. 202–7

(1987), 'Neuroimmunomodulation', in George Adelman (ed.), *Encyclopedia of Neuroscience*, Vol. II, Birkhauser, Boston, pp. 798–9

(1990), 'Neuroimmunomodulation takes off', *Immunology Today*, XI(11), pp. 381–3

Spector, Herbert Novera and Korneva, Elena A. (1981), 'Neurophysiology, immunophysiology, and neuroimmunomodulation', in Robert Ader (ed.), *Psychoneuroimmunology*, Academic Press, New York, pp. 449–74

Stewart, John and Varela, Francisco J. (1989), 'Exploring the meaning of connectivity in the immune network', *Immunological Reviews: (Copenhagen)*, CX, pp. 37–61

Temoshok, Lydia (1983), 'Emotion, adaptation, and disease: a multidimensional theory', pp. 207–233, in L. Temoshok, C. VanDyke, and L.S. Zegans (eds.), *Emotions in Health and Illness: Theoretical and Research Foundations*, Grune & Stratton, New York

Vaz, Nelson and de Faria, Ana Maria C, (1990), 'The construction of immunological identity', *Ciencia e Cultura*, XLII(7), pp. 430–44

Yates, F. Eugene (ed.) (1987), *Self-Organizing Systems: The Emergence of Order*, Plenum Press, New York

Index